Master the Art of Swimming

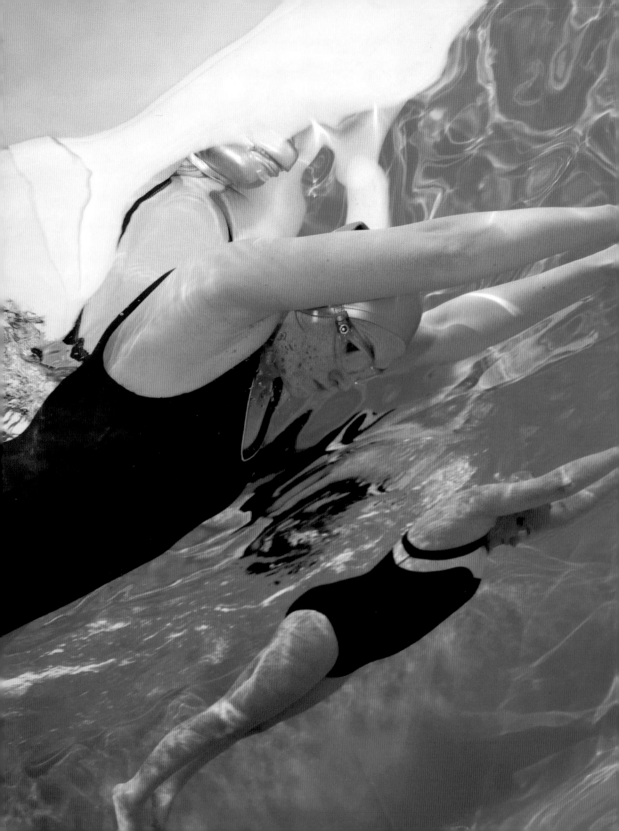

Steven Shaw

Master the Art of Swimming

Raise Your Performance with the Alexander Technique

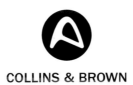

COLLINS & BROWN

First published in the United Kingdom in 2006
This edition first published in 2009 by
Collins & Brown
10 Southcombe Street
London, W14 0RA

An imprint of Anova Books Company Ltd

ISBN 978-1-84340-542-9

A CIP catalogue for this book is available from the British
Library.

10 9 8 7 6 5 4 3 2 1

Pool facilities and most photography was provided by
Graham and Yulia Parker of Swimming Pictures,
www.swimpix.com, apart from the following pages:
7, 18-19, 26-27, 80-81, 106-107, 140 Zillah Crosby
and 31, 32, 54, 55, 68, 69, 73, 74, 84, 85, 126, 127,
131, 154 Guy Hearn

Reproduction by Anorax Imaging Ltd
Printed and bound by 1010 Printing International
Limited, China

Keep updated. Email sales@anovabooks.com for FREE
email alerts on forthcoming titles.

www.anovabooks.com

Dedication

Dedicated to the memory of my great teacher Zeev
Tadmore who gave me the confidence to truly explore
my relationship with the water from an Alexander
Technique perspective.

Acknowledgments

I wish to thank my parents Helen and Maurice Shaw for
their encouragement and unwavering support. The
material in this book is the result of work over the years
and I am indebted to all of my colleagues, students and
pupils for helping me turn my passion into a career.
Particular credit goes to Charlotte Parry-Crooke,
Malcolm Balk, Philip Tibenham and Armand D'Angour.

I wish to thank Limor Shaw who is currently developing
the work in Israel, for her deep understanding and long-
term commitment to the Shaw Method. To my friend and
colleague Gillian Jordan for making it possible to train
others to teach this Method and for her help and
suggestions with the text.

I would like to thank Zillah Crosby, my life partner, for
backing me up on every stage of this project. Without her
insightful contributions and attention to detail this book
would have been infinitely inferior.

I would like to acknowledge the many people who
directly contributed to the creation of this book. Firstly to
my Publisher Katie Cowan, Commissioning Editor
Victoria Alers-Hankey, creative director Gemma Wilson
and designer Thomas Keenes – along with the rest of the
team at Anova for producing this beautifully crafted book.
To Graham, Yulia Parker, David Tozer together with Zillah
Crosby and John Paul for the excellent photography.
Thanks to Joanne Makin for her skilful illustrations.
Thanks also to the models Jennifer Evans, Vicky Harmer,
Deborah and Helen Stevens and Huseyin Dermis who
skilfully embody the Shaw Method. To Margaret and Tony
Farrell for their kindness and patience in allowing us to
use their pool in Esher. Finally thanks to Jonathon Drake
and Andrew Crosby for their assistance and suggestions
with the manuscript.

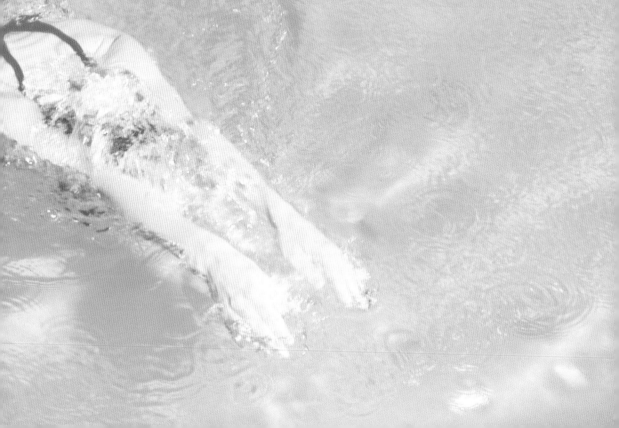

CONTENTS

IN PRAISE OF SWIMMING

An open mind, a swimming pool or stretch of calm water and this book are all you need to realize your untapped potential for freedom of movement with the Shaw Method. Prepare to embark on an amazing journey of self-discovery. In the rhythmic movements of swimming, free from the downward pressure of gravity, you can discover the ultimate form of meditation. Swimming is the supreme form of exercise for mind, body and spirit – as well as improving flexibility and tone it will also boost your self-esteem and sense of well-being. Whatever challenges you face in life, swimming always helps: when you are stressed it relaxes you, when you are exhausted it revitalizes you, and when your muscles are stiff it releases them. Forget Prozac – the remedy is in H_2O!

Exercise fads come and go, but swimming always remains at the top of the popularity charts. The psychological benefits of immersion, rather than the knowledge that swimming is good for joints and muscles, keep millions of people switched on to swimming. It is an ideal antidote to our pressured lives, offering a rare opportunity to rejuvenate the body while allowing the mind to rest.

The verb 'to swim' is defined as 'the ability to propel oneself through water', whereas the noun 'swimming' is generally defined as 'a competitive sport'. The competitive perspective is so pervasive that even the *Oxford English Dictionary* describes swimming purely in terms of being a sport. This attitude is extremely limiting. As long as you gauge your performance in the water by the number of laps you swim or whether you arrive at the end of the pool before the next person, there is little chance of discovering the riches water has to offer.

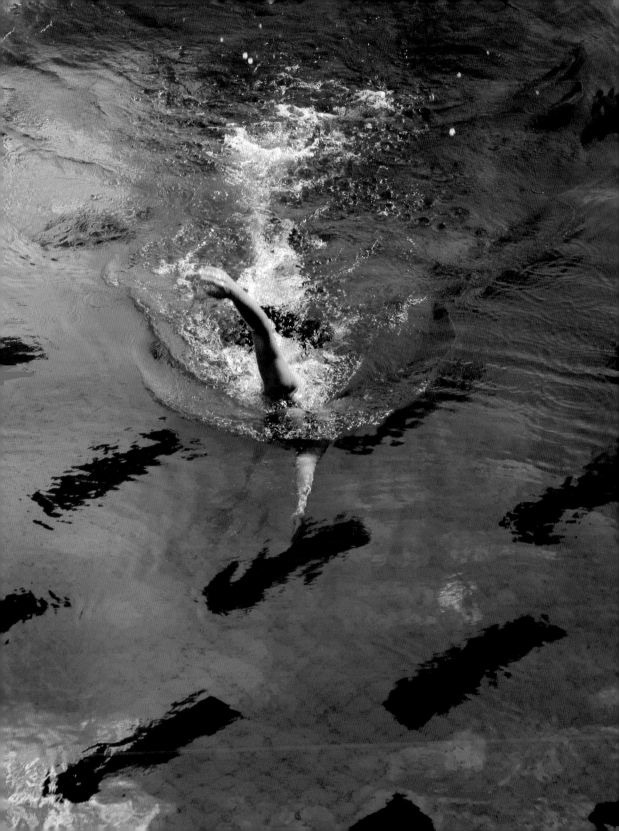

It is, however, important to acknowledge that a competitive outlook has been vital to the remarkable evolution of swimming. Without the motivation to go faster, human beings would probably still swim like other land-based mammals, using what is essentially a form of walking. Competition has led us to develop four ingenious ways of moving through the water: breaststroke, backstroke, front crawl and butterfly. Man's ability to swim well also derives from certain unique physical characteristics. Only human babies, born with subcutaneous fat, can float and swim from birth. Of all primates, only humans have a descended larynx, allowing us to easily take in air through the mouth when swimming.

What differentiates the approach outlined here from others is that it draws on the Alexander Technique. The Technique's central idea is that the relationship between head, neck and back determines the quality of the body's overall coordination. When the neck is free and the head balances lightly at the top of the spine we are able to function more efficiently; when it is tense and the vertebrae are compressed our functioning is adversely affected. My years of experience have confirmed that the head-neck-back relationship is of utmost importance and that improving this relationship is the single most significant factor affecting swimming performance.

We are now entering a new phase in the evolution of swimming. This book will help you transcend the competitive mindset and recraft each stroke to promote the optimum use of the self. This approach to swimming is closer to a martial art than a competitive sport – winning or losing are mere distractions from an ongoing journey towards self-mastery. Water is an ideal environment for self-development; it amplifies psychophysical patterns, providing the opportunity to become aware of how thoughts affect quality of movement. Swimming is unlike any other physical activity: apart from needing to coordinate the whole body in the horizontal plane, you also have to be in tune with the water. If you try hard and apply too much effort you will flounder; swimming gracefully is more about letting go and going with the flow than it is about pushing yourself.

To the evolved or enlightened swimmer, there are a number of ways of measuring one's performance. Speed is just one indicator, but no more significant than, for example, the distance travelled per stroke or the relative energy expended. A master of swimming never compromises a good body form in the quest for speed – hunching the shoulders in breaststroke reduces drag but is unacceptable as it has a detrimental effect on body alignment. This is not to say that swimming in a more mindful way reduces speed; on the contrary with the Shaw Method most people are able to swim considerably faster and further than they ever thought possible. This new approach limits the energy expended on non-propulsive movements, gaining greater purchase on the water and so realizing maximum benefit from precious time in the water.

If you are on the look out for a training manual that provides elaborate tables telling you how far and fast to swim and how much rest to take between each set, look elsewhere. There are countless 'get fit' swimming books and websites that will give you this type of information. If you are looking for something more reflective that encourages you to pause, rethink your relationship with the water and explore each stroke in depth, read on. Instead of mindlessly swimming lap after lap, you will learn to pay attention to the process of swimming and develop the quality of the experience. This learning goes far beyond the pool, providing you with a powerful new model with which to approach any activity.

Taking the plunge into learning the art of swimming may seem somewhat daunting, particularly for those with a more sedentary lifestyle. You may feel self-conscious about your size and the prospect of being seen in public in a swimming costume. However, having decided to embark on a fitness programme it is far better to begin in the pool where the effects of buoyancy significantly reduce the risks of injuring weight-bearing joints. More regular swimmers may feel self conscious about practising new strokes or performing unusual looking practices. Take comfort from the fact only those swimmers straining their necks to keep their faces out of the water will be watching. With any luck your progress will inspire them to join in!

Steven's Story

My earliest memories of swimming are of splashing around in the local open-air lido where I spent much of my leisure time. The pool never seemed to lose its magical appeal. During the summer months, the anticipation was often overwhelming. I have vivid memories of one scorching day, standing impatiently in what was surely the longest queue ever. The interminable wait added to my sense of excitement and I can remember my heart racing when my nose picked up the sweet scent of chlorine. When we finally arrived at the turnstiles, I had to be restrained from running ahead. I always wore my trunks under my trousers to avoid wasting precious time.

Until the age of eight I spent my time at the children's pool, a large semi-circular construction where water streamed from the mouths of two lion statues. The pool had a gradual, beach-style entrance with sloping sides – great fun to run in and out of when the lifeguards weren't watching! We picnicked on the grassy banks surrounding the pool and after the compulsory hour's wait to ensure digestion we raced back to the pool for more aquatic fun. The lido was much more than a pool: it was a place to hang out with friends and family.

I was a clumsy child and the pool was one of the few places I felt safe to explore movement without injuring myself. I spent hours inventing pool games. My favourite was 'The Torpedo'. The torpedo lay face down in the water and the launcher got hold of his feet and pushed him forward; whoever got the farthest was the winner. During my experience as the torpedo I discovered that by tucking in my chin and breathing out slowly I would travel further, that is as long as the launcher was any good. Handstands and underwater cartwheels were also great fun.

In hindsight, these early experiences were invaluable for cultivating a feeling of confidence and ease in the water. It was only when I started teaching adults that I began to appreciate the value of simply exploring the water.

Peer pressure and the lure of deeper water led me to the conclusion that it was time to learn to swim 'properly', so I enrolled at a local swimming class. The teacher was from the old school of teaching and if a child held back he would be forced in. The experience of witnessing these scenes made a strong impression on me. I can vividly remember the atmosphere of fear at the school and can recall thinking that there must be a better way to teach.

Time to get serious about swimming

I graduated from the local swimming school to the Mermaids and Marlins swimming club, and started to train and compete. The club had some international-level swimmers and it was inspirational to train alongside them. It was not long before I was training for four hours a day, squeezed in before and after school. Our coach drove us hard, an approach which sometimes verged on bullying. One one occasion he caught me pulling a lane rope along and punished me with a painful 1,500 metres of butterfly, which put me off the stroke for years.

I pushed myself to the limit, naively believing his axiom that 'Training is suffering; after suffering comes results.' Yet I never got beyond county level. Despite being fit and strong, my technique let me down.

For the most part, my training consisted of swimming lap after lap, and I would only occasionally get feedback from my coach. During these rare sessions he analysed my stroke and this was always useful. I yearned to swim with more finesse instead of thoughtlessly thrashing up and down the pool. I read numerous technique manuals, but although these were interesting they did not provide me with the tools to fundamentally change my way of swimming.

I achieved my best times in the breaststroke and like most competitive breaststrokers I cultivated a pattern of hunching my shoulders to achieve maximum streamlining. Looking back at photographs of myself during

Steven's Story CONTINUED

this period, it is clear that my habit of rounding my shoulders when on dry land was shaped during this period. I was oblivious to the link between the way I used my body in and out of the water.

By the age of seventeen, I was burnt out. Without success to spur me on, I no longer enjoyed training and to cap it all my neck and upper back felt sore. The feeling of freedom of movement that attracted me to swimming in the first place had disappeared. I quit swimming and vowed never to return. Giving up was a tremendous liberation: instead of spending hours every week training and travelling to and from the pool, I was able to develop a life beyond swimming.

The Alexander Technique

I became interested in political theory and went to study Philosophy and Politics at Manchester University, in England. I was particularly interested in exploring the connection between thought and action.

Like many students, I did very little physical activity, and my poor posture combined with the pressure of exams caused my back and neck to deteriorate. I tried massage, osteopathy and acupuncture, which temporarily alleviated the discomfort but did not bring lasting relief. A friend suggested that I try the Alexander Technique (AT), a system of postural re-education. He explained that it addresses the root causes of habitual patterns. I was sceptical but my friend was clearly benefiting from it – he moved with a new sense of poise and appeared to be more at ease with himself.

Eventually I signed up for a series of weekly private lessons. They were no immediate panacea. The lessons were challenging and it was several months before I noticed any changes. We explored simple activities such as standing and walking. The teacher demonstrated *Primary Control* – a dynamic relationship between the head, neck and back, which is at the core of the Alexander approach. I came to the daunting realization that most of the time I was completely oblivious to the way I moved and functioned. However, what was liberating about these early lessons (in contrast to my swimming training) was that I never felt criticized or judged. My teacher simply encouraged me to direct my attention away from trying to do the right thing and instead towards working on eliminating bad habits. It was the cumulative effect of letting my neck be free so that my back lengthened and widened, and the notion of taking responsibility for my own condition, which inspired me to train further in the Technique.

In 1987 I began a three-year Alexander Technique teacher-training course in Tel Aviv. In Israel the AT is a widely accepted method for re-educating the body, and is a part of basic training for military pilots. The head of training at the school, Zeev Tadmore, came from a sporting and martial arts background.

A central element of AT training is that before working with others you are expected to employ the principles of the AT yourself. The psychophysical state in which I arrived at the school was not a good one. My posture was still poor, and my shoulders and upper back constantly ached. My teacher was always positive and created a supportive and nurturing environment. He encouraged me to investigate the sources of my poor alignment, which included swimming.

During my time in Israel I worked as a lifeguard, which gave me the opportunity to swim again. After an absence of five years it was good to reconnect with the water; however, a familiar aching sensation in my neck confirmed that my poor posture and what the AT describes as 'misuse' of the body were linked to my years of competitive training. The focus in those years had been purely on speed with little regard for my overall well-being.

My inability to notice the build-up of tension in my body when swimming, despite being an AT student, was particularly distressing.

Steven's Story CONTINUED

This lack of awareness was hard to comprehend, but my teacher explained that habitual patterns of behaviour normally feel right and to change them frequently feels wrong. For me, the tension was so familiar that it felt natural, whereas swimming without strain felt odd and even incorrect. As soon as I got into the water my old, habitual ways of swimming returned: in breaststroke my shoulders ended up by my ears and despite attempting to swim slowly and mindfully, I couldn't stop myself from racing whenever a fast swimmer came near me. I began to realize that the postural patterns I had developed in the water were merely symptoms of a much more complex problem which concerned my whole approach to swimming.

Gradually, as my body awareness developed, I began to move more easily through the water. It was still difficult to get into the pool without a fixed goal, however, such as completing a certain number of lengths in a given time. But by controlling my tendency to rush, in all aspects of my life as well as in the water, I was able to alter the way I swam. I began to appreciate that water offered both a sense of stillness and a unique opportunity to explore freedom of movement.

When I began exploring my relationship with water, I was surprised by the variety and intensity of surfacing memories. Keeping a journal covering the content of my practice sessions and related thoughts and feelings helped me absorb the significance of this process and provided a useful record of my journey. I now encourage my pupils to keep a similar record whilst the experiences are still fresh in their mind, which many find similarly helpful.

Working with others
Apart from improving my own relationship with the water during this time, my job as a lifeguard gave me ample opportunity to observe others swimming. I was shocked by the number of people who swam with their

heads held up out of the water, and from my new Alexander perspective could now see how much neck strain this was causing. I began to notice those who swam in a graceful, almost effortless way, allowing the head and neck to move freely in and out of the water. I became increasingly aware that the principal elements that set a good swimmer apart lay in the relationship between the head, neck and back. Poorer swimmers pulled their heads back and fixed their neck muscles.

A job at a holiday resort gave me a chance to discover more about people's early experiences of swimming. I was struck by the number of adults who recalled negative incidents. They almost always reported that their teachers, like mine, had encouraged them to apply more effort in order to swim better. Together with my then wife Limor, also an AT trainee, I began to explore ways of using hands-on guidance to help them feel more comfortable in the water. Initially I worked mainly with fearful swimmers, but found that competent swimmers also benefited from this approach.

In 1992, a year after completing the AT teacher training, I returned to the UK and began teaching the Technique in London. I also completed a couple of swimming teacher courses at the local pool. I enjoyed the courses greatly, but was very surprised that you were not required to swim and were not allowed to teach from within the water.

Through conversations with my AT pupils I found that many of them swam with their faces out of the water so I decided to offer 'water confidence' lessons and within a relatively short time I was teaching a range of abilities. I learned a great deal through my interaction with these pupils. I could see that the combination of my competitive swimming experience and the Alexander training was of enormous value.

In 1994, a pupil who was to have a major impact on my work booked a series of swimming lessons. Armand D'Angour was in his mid-30s and wanted to overcome a fear of water. He had tried to learn to swim several

Steven's Story CONTINUED

times, but with little success. He had taken lessons in the Alexander Technique and was intrigued by the prospect of applying AT principles to swimming. The difference between his lessons with me and all his previous instruction was the fact that I was successfully able to redirect his attention and instead of fighting the water he learned to enjoy it. Armand quickly learnt to swim with confidence and ease. He was delighted with his progress and we decided to write a book together to inspire others to learn to swim.

In 1996, *The Art of Swimming: a New Direction with the Alexander Technique* was published by Ashgrove Press, offering a clear alternative to the traditional model of swimming. It was the first book written from an Alexander Technique standpoint to make an in-depth philosophical investigation into a sporting activity. It challenged the popular belief that swimming is always beneficial, illustrating how a defective style can do more harm than good. It urged people to stop striving to swim faster and further and start swimming in a more mindful way. The book received an unexpected level of media attention and became a bestseller in its field.

The Shaw Method

The *Art of Swimming* not only had an impact on swimmers far and wide, it also dramatically affected my life. Overnight, the demand for lessons became overwhelming. I wanted to establish a teacher-training programme, but was hesitant to define my way of teaching as a method because I feared this would hinder the flexibility and intuitive nature of the teaching process. However, without a clearly defined and structured teaching model the approach could not be passed on to other teachers, severely limiting its potential growth. So, after much deliberation, I began to formalize the teaching as the Shaw Method of Swimming. Looking back, this was a seminal moment in the development of the work and had a very positive impact on both my teaching and swimming.

Although I had been endeavouring to apply Alexander Technique principles to swimming, and had discovered new ways of guiding and supporting people in the water, the work was still in its infancy. It had not yet been formulated as a comprehensive teaching method.

Using a camcorder, I investigated my own swimming style to find out whether I was moving in a way that promoted the best possible use of myself. I remembered that Alexander had gone through a similar process himself with the use of mirrors. Seeing myself swim for the first time was quite an alarming and humbling experience. My head was much higher than I thought it ought to be and although my movement looked fluent, my arm and leg actions were not symmetrical. I concluded that my swimming style required a complete overhaul.

From my AT experience I knew that to try and eliminate faults whilst performing the full stroke was unlikely to be successful, as the stimulus to move in habitual ways would just be too strong. I reasoned that the best course of action was to separate out the core elements of each stroke and work on them in isolation – both in the water and on dry land. Hopefully this would override strongly ingrained patterns and offer a real possibility of producing a new way of moving. The approach worked and proved to be a powerful way of rebuilding my strokes; it also produced positive side effects, altering the way I felt and moved both in and out of the pool. Having found a way of fundamentally changing my swimming technique, I now had the beginnings of a new model with which to teach others.

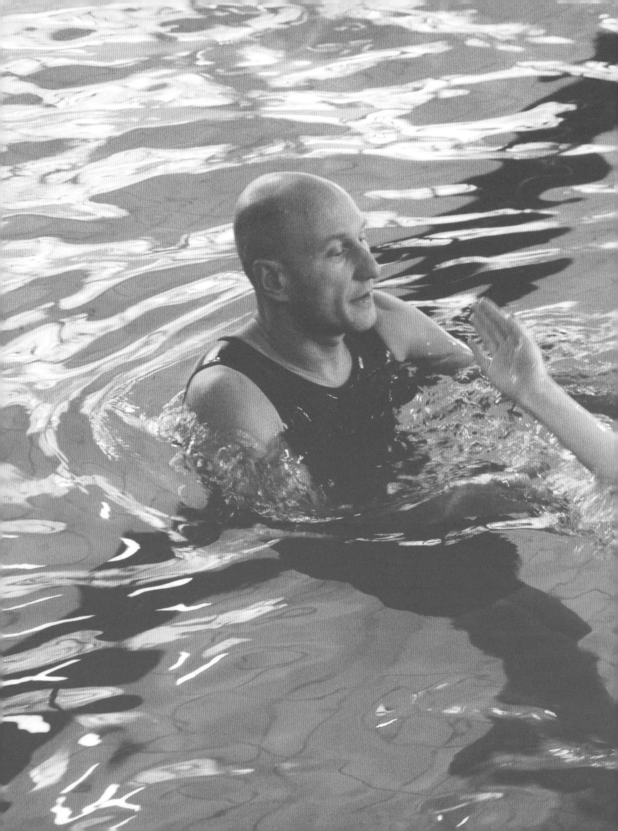

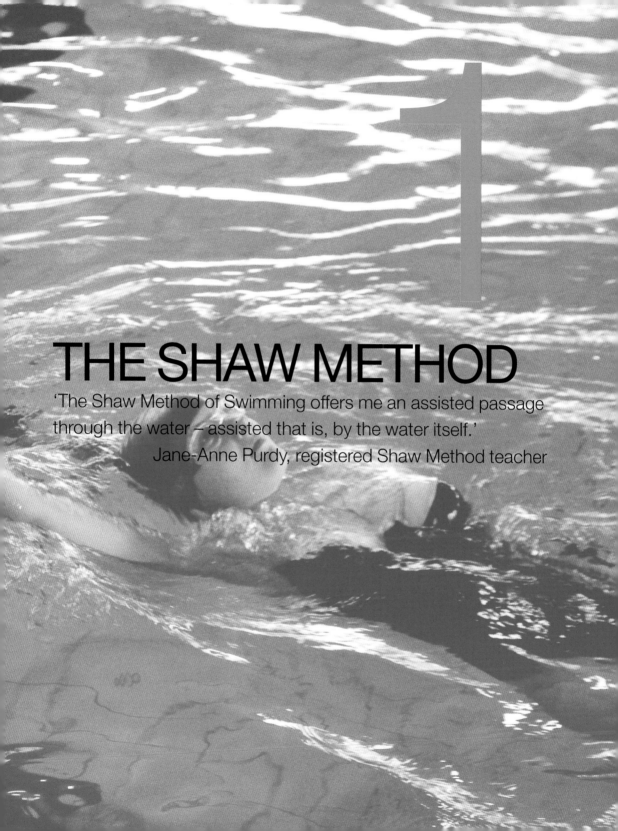

1

THE SHAW METHOD

'The Shaw Method of Swimming offers me an assisted passage through the water – assisted that is, by the water itself.'
Jane-Anne Purdy, registered Shaw Method teacher

Although swimming is one of the most popular forms of exercise, most people do not swim well enough to really benefit from the time they spend in the water, and many have developed styles that strain their joints. The underlying goals of speed and competition at the heart of conventional swimming instruction often impede the acquisition of vital skills. Few are able to swim continuously for 20 minutes – which is generally considered the minimum time to gain cardiovascular benefit.

Learning the Shaw Method

If you have picked up this book you are probably fed up with thrashing around in the pool or bored with counting laps. Let the Shaw Method start a new era in your relationship with water.

This chapter explains the key principles of the Shaw Method of Swimming and dispels myths and fallacies. Chapter 2 guides you though a series of practices that teach the core elements of the Method. These preliminary practices may appear too pedestrian for more accomplished swimmers. However, the basics of awareness, direction and balance are at the heart of a good stroke and must be mastered to develop the repertoire of aquatic skills required for a healthier and more pleasurable style of swimming.

Chapters 3–6 guide you though a series of easy-to-follow, progressive practices on land and in the water, which teach my unique formula for developing the four strokes: front crawl, breaststroke, back crawl and butterfly. You will discover that a non-propulsive movement precedes every propulsive movement. These chapters also include accounts of each stroke's relative health benefits, outlining not only what to do but, just as importantly, what to avoid. It is beneficial to work through these with a partner as well as by yourself.

This book is not a 'quick fix' to your aquatic woes; rather it points the way towards a more mindful and conscious relationship with water. Goals such as improving cardiovascular fitness must be temporarily set aside until you have established a firm foundation for your swimming strokes. Thereafter you will be in a position to obtain greater health and fitness benefits from your time in the water.

The key to success is cultivating a positive, open approach to learning. Your level of skill or expertise in the water when you begin this journey is immaterial. Free yourself from the pressure of trying to perform the practices 'correctly' and use them to start exploring the unknown. I have found that those most successful at mastering the art of swimming posses the ability to stop, listen and be patient.

When you flick through this book, the sheer number of practices may overwhelm you. Don't follow them mechanically – they are there to encourage you to experiment with the way you think and move, heighten your awareness and inspire creativity. It is unnecessary to memorize exact sequences or the finer points of a particular practice; a deeper understanding will come with time. Initially, it is important to grasp the main purpose of a practice and how it may apply to you.

It is futile to be overly concerned with stroke mechanics before you feel at home in the water. Learn to trust the water and allow it to support you instead of struggling against it. This will completely transform the experience of swimming. This may sound obvious, yet most swimmers find it hard to truly relax in the water.

Swimming with the Alexander Technique

The Shaw Method is a creative step-by-step approach that has helped thousands of people of all ages and abilities transform their experience of swimming. In contrast with the majority of teachers who adopt a competitive perspective, the Shaw Method draws its inspiration from F.M Alexander's powerful technique for rediscovering natural balance and poise. Brief descriptions of Alexander's principles follow. Please thoroughly acquaint yourself with them as they are used throughout this book.

Use – A term to describe a person's psychophysical interaction with their environment. Swimming with good use involves moving through the water in a way that promotes good alignment with minimal physical or mental strain.

Primary Control – For Alexander the quality of the head-neck-back relationship was the single most important factor affecting overall use. Paying attention to form and allowing the head to lead the rest of the body is the best way to resolve specific stroke faults.

Giving directions – The ability to project a series of constructive thoughts that promote lengthening and widening. In swimming to counter the tendency of pulling the arms backwards it is useful to direct your attention to holding the water and moving the torso forward.

Kinaesthetic awareness – The ability to sense the position, orientation and movement of the body. Feedback from the water enhances the development of body awareness.

End Gaining – Striving for results without attending to process. Swimming for fitness without considering technique often leads to strain and injury.

Inhibition – Creating the space for choice between stimulus and reaction. To counter the undesirable habit of taking a big breath before putting the face in the water it is necessary to inhibit this automatic response before consciously inhaling.

Faulty sensory appreciation – Good use requires accurate kinaesthetic awareness. Force of habit and a lack of conscious control undermine this ability leading to faulty sensory appreciation. If you are accustomed to an uneven breaststroke leg action a symmetrical leg action is likely to feel wrong.

Thinking in Activity – Swimming in an unthinking way reduces the ability to feel and respond to water, a mindful approach enables you to become more responsive to the effects of buoyancy and resistance and thereby more in tune with the water.

Non-doing – The conscious ability to leave oneself alone and avoid automatic responses. It is preferable to consciously let go and allow the water to support you as opposed to trying to hold yourself up.

Startle response – An automatic response to an unexpected, sudden stimulus, our head reflexively moves back and down, compressing the neck and stressing the rest of the body. While the startle response is a natural reaction to fear, it is inappropriate in the water and has a detrimental affect on the ability to swim comfortably. Learning to free the neck and allowing our back its full length and width promotes calmness and ease in the water.

The power of habit

I am often taken aback by some people's unrealistic expectations of the learning process. Swimming habits develop over many years and it is naive to expect an instant transformation. Tai chi masters consider that it takes around 500 repetitions to learn a new movement and 5,000 to re-pattern an old one.

Everyone has a tendency to return to habitual patterns in the water. The sooner you learn to recognize these patterns, the quicker you can start the process of changing them. Don't give yourself a hard time when you revert to your old ways and don't expect instant results; you will make progress.

Because our neuromuscular system is designed to work in concert with gravity you may find some of the instructions counterintuitive. To swim effectively you really have to use your brain; following your instincts and doing what comes naturally is unlikely to produce good results.

Over-breathing is one of the most common and unhelpful aquatic habits. Most people unnecessarily and automatically swallow excessive quantities of air just before submerging their faces. They are oblivious to this pattern. Do you do this? Can you choose a more appropriate course of action and inhale passively?

Unless you concentrate, you are likely to slip back into the unconscious pattern.

The power of an ingrained habit also makes it more difficult to correct stroke faults than you might envisage. Because the pattern has been repeated so many times, it feels normal and comfortable. Also, the root cause of a particular pattern may be far from obvious, as the following example from my own experience indicates.

On seeing footage of my front crawl, I was concerned to note that my left and right above-water arm actions were different. I could see that my left hand twisted as it entered the water, which surprised me as I am left-handed and expected to have more control with the left hand than the right. For several months, I focused attention on my left arm to rectify this, but disappointingly the action remained virtually unchanged. It was only when someone pointed out that my left arm looked more effective underwater that I began to unravel this puzzle. I finally grasped the fact that the over-rotation of my left arm resulted from a less than effective underwater action of the right arm. This experience taught me that the process of remedying a particular stroke fault involves three essential stages: an awareness of what is actually happening, an accurate appreciation of the root cause of the difficulty, and a clear psychophysical strategy for change.

Stillness and movement

Learning the art of swimming requires a major shift in your approach to movement in water and on land. Stillness, and being in the moment, are the starting points for all conscious movement. To perform a sequence of movements accurately, it is necessary to have a clear idea of the desired objective. Pause and think before launching into any of the practices: you are more likely to achieve positive results with appropriate preparation. Many people find it extremely useful to visualize a sequence of movements, at the correct pace, before proceeding.

When pupils perform a movement incorrectly, I ask them to describe what they were attempting to do. This often reveals that they were either performing the wrong action or were simply not thinking at all. Allowing the mind to wander, as Alexander pointed out, is a major impediment to developing body awareness.

Where to swim

It is important to select a suitable environment in which to practise. Ideally, this should be a warm pool with a large area of shallow water. Try to avoid crowded, deep or cold pools. A teaching pool at the local leisure centre may be a good option. If you cannot get regular access to an ideal environment, make the best of what is available. The great thing about the practices in this book is that they do not require a large area of water. Working within a smaller area can be an advantage; you are required to stop more often, helping you to pay attention moment to moment.

Pool temperature is potentially one of the most challenging issues for anyone learning the Shaw Method. An average pool is 27–29°C (80–84°F), which feels comfortable if you are swimming laps, but if you are less confident or working through some of the less energetic sequences in this book, it can feel very chilly. If you start to feel too cold, include some more vigorous movements or shorten the session. Alternatively, you could wear a swimming cap as you lose around 30 per cent of your body heat from the top of your head; if you are particularly susceptible to the cold, why not try a lightweight thermal swimming top.

The Art of Swimming on dry land

For many of the water-based practices, there are equivalent ones to do on dry land. These are an integral part of the Shaw Method and should not be viewed as unnecessary or superfluous to the process of swimming. They help establish and reinforce new patterns of movement in preparation for swimming, developing your kinaesthetic awareness and sense of balance and control. You may initially find it hard to relate the land practices (which for the most part are performed upright) to swimming movements, but with regular repetition the link will become clearer.

Many pupils are surprised to find that seemingly complex movements are more easily absorbed and integrated into their swimming through regular land work. Some people feel self-conscious about performing swimming movements out of the water. If your friends or family think you have a screw loose, tell them it is a new martial art! Spend just a few minutes a day and it will not be long before you start reaping the benefits.

Our swimming habits can be so strong that it is often easier to change the tone and quality of the movements simply by stepping out of the water. The effects of buoyancy and resistance obviously make working on land a very different experience to working in water. However, on land you can develop the desired sequences of movements and repeat them often enough for them to feel familiar.

Practice sessions

Initially, try to spend 20–30 minutes on each session. When you are more experienced, you will be able to centre your attention for longer periods. Work on no more than four new practices in any one session. As discussed earlier, even the most elementary practices take a while to master, and until the new pattern of movement is firmly established the old, habitual one is likely to creep back. Avoid the temptation to swim the full stroke during the early stages, as this is likely to reinforce old patterns and leave you confused.

Working with a partner

Compared to other health and fitness pursuits, swimming can feel quite solitary. For some this provides the privacy that they lack in other parts of their lives; others may welcome the opportunity to share the experience.

In the absence of a Shaw Method teacher, partner work is excellent for developing awareness, with a great deal to be learned through mutual observation and feedback. You may be surprised by how quickly your observation skills grow. Be sensitive towards your partner and always give constructive feedback without overly focusing on what you think he or she is doing wrong.

Myths about swimming and fitness

It is not necessarily the case that practice makes perfect – it can make things worse. Many regular swimmers rehearse the same mistakes; bad habits become more ingrained and harder to unlearn. It is imperative to practise in a constructive way and think about the quality of movement.

Believing that if something does not work at first you should try harder is often a formula for failure rather than success. It is more productive to approach swimming with a spirit of exploration.

You do not need to wear yourself out in order to have a worthwhile workout. A healthy approach to fitness requires good body alignment and a good technique. Many people underestimate the importance of this and think they can improve their swimming by just getting fitter. What usually happens is that they get more efficient at injuring themselves! Put aerobic fitness objectives to one side until you have established a healthy way of swimming.

Some people are under the impression that they do not need to think about the way they swim. They use swimming as a way of switching off and let their minds wander. However, if you do not pay attention to the way you are swimming you are not only more likely to injure yourself, but your mind is more likely to drift to things that bother you. Paying attention to what you are doing is a better way of switching off, as it clears the mind of its usual chatter.

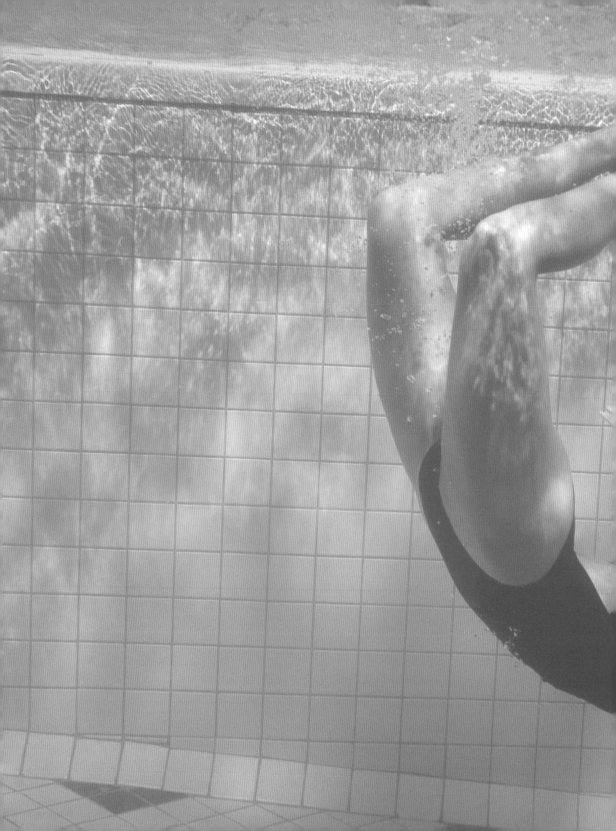

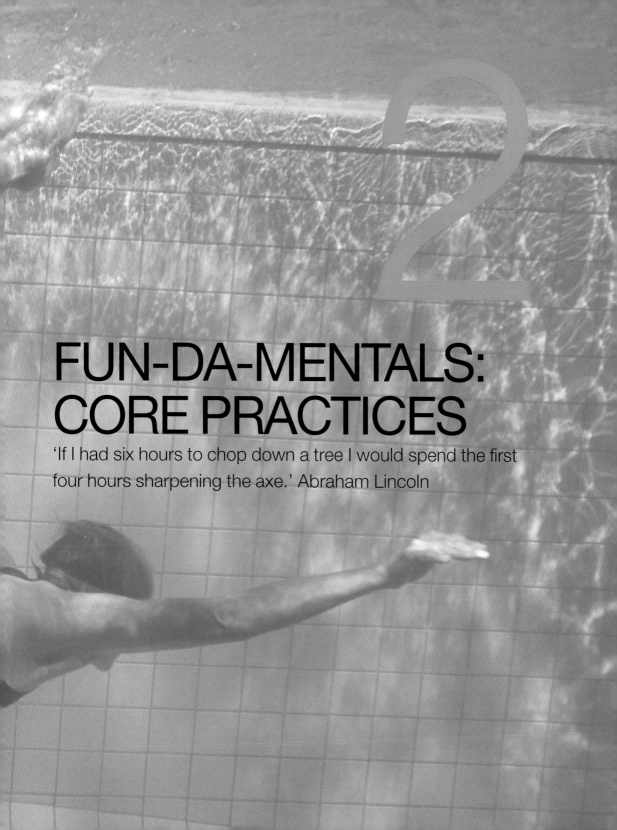

FUN-DA-MENTALS: CORE PRACTICES

'If I had six hours to chop down a tree I would spend the first four hours sharpening the axe.' Abraham Lincoln

Back to basics

The title of this chapter, 'Fun-da-mentals', emphasizes the fact that it is more fun to be imaginative and mindful in the water than to switch off and swim on automatic pilot. This section guides you through a series of foundation practices that will help you to explore and understand the physics of swimming, particularly the effects of buoyancy and resistance. If you are an accomplished swimmer, do not think that you can skip this section. Whatever your ability, you have to go 'back to basics'. In order to develop a way of swimming that promotes the best possible 'use' of the body, as the Alexander Technique describes it, you must have a wide repertoire of skills. Although many of these skills can be cultivated during the process of re-learning the four strokes, they are more effectively assimilated without the distraction of trying to get from one end of the pool to the other.

Here is an opportunity to develop a new relationship with the water. The practices in this chapter enhance awareness of the body, poise and balance, enabling you to stop struggling against the water and start working with it. They not only offer a solid base for swimming more effectively but are also beneficial in themselves, improving overall poise and balance on dry land.

Buoyancy

On land, gravitational force exerts a downward pressure on our bodies, which causes compression of weight-bearing joints including the spine, ankles, knees and hips. On entering the water, we are instantly liberated from these downward pressures because water counteracts the effect of gravity. When the body is submerged, the effects of buoyancy create more space for the joints to move, so instead of joints being wedged together they gently float apart. When submerged to chest level, the upward pressure of the water effectively reduces body weight by 90 per cent, allowing movement with minimal strain on the joints and ligaments. Leonardo Da Vinci wrote that swimming is the closest Man will ever get to the sensation of flying.

The capacity of an object to float is determined by its relative density or its weight and the amount of water it displaces. If the amount of water displaced weighs more than the object, the object will float; if the water weighs less than it, the object will sink. In other words, for an object to sink, the force of gravity must be greater than that of the upthrust produced by the water.

The average density of the human body is a little less than that of fresh water, which means that in a typical swimming pool most people float naturally.

In the sea or in a floatation tank, where the water has a much greater density, the body floats higher in the water.

Our ability to float is also influenced by body type: a lean, muscular person will usually find it more difficult to float than someone who is more rounded. The muscle mass to body fat ratio is the main reason why older people find it easier to float. Over the age of forty, most people tend to lose muscle tone and gain body fat, which is why people who tended to sink in their youth often discover that it is much easier to float when they reach middle age. Another factor that significantly affects buoyancy is muscular tension. This is particularly apparent in apprehensive swimmers, who tend to swim with contracted muscles. By developing the ability to release and lengthen, even those with a higher propensity to sink can discover how to optimize the effects of buoyancy and become accomplished swimmers.

Balance and stability

One of the hallmarks of an efficient swimmer is the ability to achieve a horizontal body position. Although most people can float, few can do so horizontally. The centre of buoyancy is located in the upper torso, due to the concentration of air in the lungs, whereas the centre of mass is in the relatively heavy hip area. The natural tendency of the upper body to float and the lower body to sink makes the finding of a relatively flat position in the water far from straightforward. It helps to 'let go' and allow the water to support you; however, unless you are extremely buoyant, your legs will still tend to drag you down. The gliding practices in this chapter will teach you how to achieve a horizontal position by fine-tuning the alignment of the head and the direction of the limbs.

Although the ability to float in a relatively static situation is an important skill, maintaining balance in a more dynamic situation, when arms and legs are producing propulsion, is even more critical. Efficient swimmers constantly adjust their balance to maintain stability. In the crawl, for example, the left arm counter-balances the action of the right leg.

The relative weight of the head in relation to the rest of the body means that its position is vital. If you lie horizontally in the water with your face submerged, you can immediately detect how ostensibly minute sideways movements of the head influence the rest of the body. In water, where the head acts as a rudder leading the way, the significance of a good head-neck-back relationship is amplified. An awareness of this not only improves poise when swimming, but can also promote a greater understanding of the profound effect that the carriage of the head has on everyday life. It is useful to explore this phenomenon, as by raising awareness of your head-neck-back relationship on dry land, you will find it easier to maintain primary control in the water.

Resistance

Another factor that differentiates movement in water and on land relates to the effects of resistance or, more accurately, hydrostatic pressure, which is around a thousand times greater in water than in air. This pressure, apart from slowing us down, gives the nervous system useful feedback and is one of the reasons why hydrotherapy is so effective in the treatment of neurological conditions. The late Christopher Reeve, who became quadriplegic following a serious riding accident, countered commonly held beliefs about his condition when he discovered that he could partially move his legs in water.

Hydrostatic pressure increases with the

depth of the water. Gently exhale and allow your body to sink, and you will notice an increase in the pressure on your ears. Place your hand just beneath the surface of the water and swish it back and forth: see how easy it is to move your hand. Now reach deeper and perform the same action: you will observe that it takes significantly more effort to produce the same movement. Hydrostatic pressure not only affects the functioning of our nervous system and limbs, but also the functioning of our internal organs, in particular the kidneys. Breathing while submersed in shoulder-deep water requires more effort than breathing on land, because the pressure of the water resists expansion of the chest.

Efficient swimming

The challenges faced by anyone wishing to master the art of swimming are to utilize the resistance of water in order to achieve maximum power without undue strain, and to become streamlined without compromising 'use'. This section points the way to meeting these challenges effectively by applying some general principles; stroke-specific guidance will be explored later.

Most people's approach to swimming is automatic; they have little appreciation of how to maximize benefit from energy expended. When they feel like going faster, they simply move their arms and legs faster and apply more effort to the whole stroke. This is counterproductive, as it not only produces strain and fatigue but also creates turbulence and increases resistance. Instead of conserving their energy on the non-propulsive parts of the stroke, they apply maximum force throughout.

The realization that a non-propulsive movement precedes each propulsive movement can completely transform their experience. Increased sensitivity and control in the non-propulsive phases enable a swimmer to find the optimum limb position before applying force, resulting in improved purchase, economy of energy and increased flow.

Alexander's notion of 'good use' provides us with a very effective barometer for assessing stroke mechanics. Ask yourself whether you are lengthening and widening your back or narrowing and shortening it. If the former is the case, this is worth cultivating; if the opposite is true, it is time to change. This contrasts greatly with a competitive approach, where speed is the goal and swimmers are encouraged to be as streamlined as possible with little regard for what constitutes good overall use. In the Shaw Method, the mark of a truly efficient swimmer is characterized by the ability to maximize distance per stroke in a way that promotes the best possible use.

Breathing with ease

The ability to breathe with ease is another major challenge for anyone wishing to master the art of swimming. An understanding of the principles of aquatic breathing will help swimmers of all abilities: confident swimmers learn to negotiate the transition between water and air without straining their necks, and less accomplished swimmers learn to approach the breathing process with less anxiety.

You will not progress with the Shaw Method unless you are able to immerse your face and breathe out calmly; the quality of the out-breath significantly affects the ability to breathe in and vice versa. Anxiety about taking in water makes many people delay inhalation for as long as possible, which only exacerbates the problem. Starved of oxygen, they feel compelled to inhale forcefully, which leads to the unpleasant sensations of either swallowing or sniffing water along with air.

Avoid getting to the point of having to take a breath: it is better to breathe out gently or inhale more frequently. Efficient swimmers time their inhalations through choice rather than necessity. Some good advice, which is drawn directly from the Alexander Technique, is to pay attention to the out-breath and allow the in-breath to happen by itself. The following points 1–7, supported by land-based practices and observation, will prepare you for a more comfortable and controlled experience of breathing in the water.

1. Breathing and primary control

More than a century ago Alexander observed that the relationship between the head, neck and back profoundly affects the respiratory system, and that whenever this relationship is out of balance, breathing is disturbed. He concluded that working on one's poise is more likely to have a positive effect than doing breathing exercises. This principle applies equally to swimming. The following practice illustrates how poor alignment has a detrimental effect on the quality of exhalation, underlining why swimming with the head pulled back reduces one's ability to breathe with ease.

- Sit forward on a stable chair with both feet firmly on the floor. Rock forward from the hips, maintaining the length of the neck and back, until your upper body is at 45° with the eyes looking forward and down (1a).
- Gently say 'Aah' and see how long you can comfortably sustain this sound.
- Now, without altering your position, take a breath in and pull the head back so your eyes look ahead. Say 'Aah' again, and note any changes in the duration or quality of the sound (1b, see overleaf). Most people experience a deterioration in tone, because their breathing apparatus is strained.

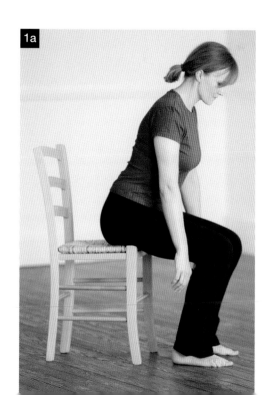

1a

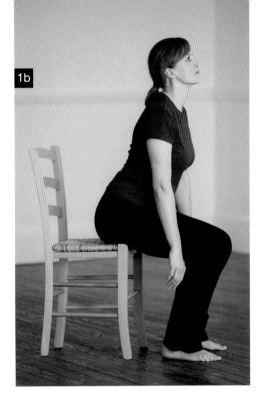

1b

2. Oral inhalation

Inhalation through the nose is all right when breathing on land, but inappropriate when swimming. When you raise your face after being submerged, the nostrils remain moist and so if you breathe in through your nose, water is likely to get drawn up the nasal passage. This unpleasant experience often leads to apprehension about submerging the face.

- Before you practise breathing when in the pool, familiarize yourself with oral inhalation out of the water.
- While breathing through the mouth, explore activities such as sitting and standing, or walking.

3. Passive inhalation

The first and most important rule of breathing with ease is to *never take a breath*! Be careful not to misinterpret this statement. I do not advocate breath-holding, but propose that passive inhalation is all that is required to swim efficiently. Excessive inhalation is unnecessary and can be harmful, leading to hyperventilation and even panic. This deeply ingrained tendency is widespread. Observe swimmers of all levels and you will see the vast majority gulping in large quantities of air in preparation for launching off. They behave as if they were about to travel a vast distance under the water or take their last breath.

4. Perils of excessive exhalation

Just as holding the breath is inadvisable, so too is the opposite pattern of explosively breathing out. Emptying your lungs completely before breathing in is not only a recipe for anxiety but also reduces buoyancy. *Trickle breathing* – exhaling gradually in the water – is a more positive alternative. Initially you may find it helpful to vocalize while breathing out.

- Explore emptying your lungs forcefully and notice how this leads to gasping.
- Now breathe out in a gentler manner and note how the resulting inhalation is calmer.
- Remember to avoid excessive or premature exhalations!

5. The oral and nasal seal

The sight of people holding their nose and breath as they prepare to put their face in the water is all too familiar. Many falsely believe that an open nose and mouth will inevitably lead to water entering the lungs. In fact, when the face is immersed, the pressure inside the lungs automatically equalizes with that of the water, producing a seal that prevents water passing the larynx. As long as you do not inhale, you can relax the nose and leave the mouth open without drawing in water. Knowledge of these oral and nasal seals can be extremely liberating for those keen to relax their breathing. The following practice, using a basin or bowl of tepid water, demonstrates this phenomenon.

- Open your mouth and gently breathe in through it.
- Maintaining an open mouth, relax the jaw and tongue, and immerse the face.
- Remain in this position for around ten seconds, without breathing.
- Enjoy the sensation of water being inside the mouth and nostrils without flooding the lungs.

6. Breathing against resistance

Many vastly underestimate the length of time they can comfortably exhale into the water. Almost as soon as they start breathing out, they feel the air in their lungs has been expended. In reality, water is much denser than air and a breath actually lasts significantly longer. Even if you play a wind instrument, you would struggle to empty your lungs in a few seconds under water.

- To simulate the effects of water pressure on breathing, place your palm over your mouth and breathe out into it. Notice how long you are able to maintain the out-breath.
- Now repeat the same action with the face unobstructed, and notice how much more quickly the breath is expelled.

7. Facial tension and breath control

On one of your field trips to the local pool, observe people's facial expressions. You may be surprised to see many people grimace just before putting their faces in the water. If you were to watch them beneath the surface, you would see that many maintain this facial tension whilst submerged. Apart from not being very flattering, this significantly impedes effective breath control. The link between respiration and facial expression is highlighted in the following practice.

- Screw up your face and attempt to say 'Aah' for a few seconds. Notice the tone and the quality of the out-breath.
- Now contrast this with a relaxed facial expression.
- Obviously, almost everyone finds it easier to exhale when the face is relaxed.

Steps in the water

You are now ready to explore the aquatic environment and start applying control to your movements. The following practices will help you to release tight muscles, achieve balance and stability, breathe with ease, generally feel more at home in the water and, most importantly, to have fun using your brain!

The opening stance for all pool-based practices, unless otherwise stated, is as follows. Stand in chest-deep water with your feet hip-width apart and your weight evenly distributed. Keep your shoulders relaxed, with your arms hanging by your sides. Look straight ahead without fixing the gaze (pictured right).

When doing the practices, soften your joints, allowing them to be movable, and experiment with breathing through the mouth. For any backward or sideways practices, look around to ensure that there is a clear pathway.

1. Weightless walking

Because walking is such a familiar, everyday activity, most people rarely pay much attention to it. It is only when injured, or trying on a new pair of shoes, that they consider how they walk. In regular walking, the arms naturally swing alternately to the legs; this cross-pattern action provides balance and stability. In water, the effects of resistance and buoyancy change the walking experience. The arms do not swing naturally; many hold them stiffly or move right leg and right arm together. In water it is not necessary to actively lift the foot: simply release the knee and allow it to float upwards, then actively put the foot down. Walking in water is an ideal way to work on balance and to acclimatize to the water, and because of the effects of resistance, it requires more energy expenditure so you can use the practice to burn calories. It is also beneficial for those with joint pain who may experience difficulty walking on dry land, as a means of re-establishing a normal walking pattern.

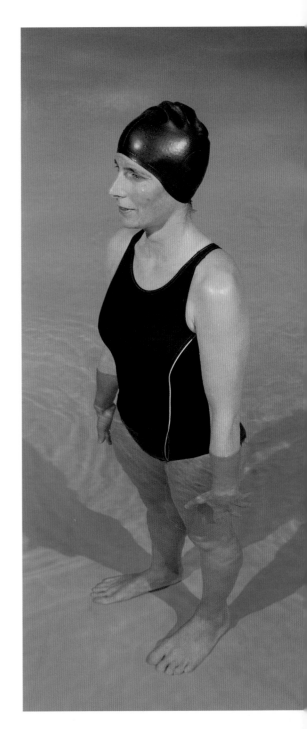

STEPS IN THE WATER

Name of Practice	Objectives
1 Weightless walking (page 34)	Acclimatizing to being in water. Working with the effects of buoyancy and resistance to achieve stability.
2 Retro walking (page 36)	Learning to ground yourself and connect to your back. An antidote to moving forward and collapsing.
3 The bellows (page 37)	Finding a streamlined path through the water. Learning to use buoyancy to widen and lengthen the back. Coordinating breathing with arm movement.
4 The lunge (page 39)	Preparing to move from the vertical to the horizontal plane. Establishing good body alignment, connecting the arms with the back.
5 Facing the water (page 40)	Understanding how our breathing apparatus is influenced by facial tension.
6 Lunging with the face submerged (page 41)	Combining balance with breath control. Remember to avoid excessive or premature exhalations.
7 The glide (see page 42)	Achieving a stable position in the water. Regaining the feet in a way that strengthens, rather than strains, the neck and back.
8 Floating on the back (see page 44)	Learning to let go while floating on the back. Lengthening and widening, and regaining the feet with poise and control.
9 Rotation (see page 46)	Developing the ability to rotate from back to front, which also aids oral and nasal breath control.
10 The wave (see page 47)	Mobilizing the whole body. Leading down with the head against the effects of buoyancy and experiencing upthrust; exploring different depths.

- Take up the opening stance. The water's buoyancy will help you to stand tall. Raise the right leg by shifting your weight on to the left leg; ensure that the knee does not go too high as this may cause a loss of balance.
- Maintaining the position of the head, make a small step forward with the left leg, and simultaneously move the right arm a few inches forward to counterbalance the leg.
- Actively press the left foot down so that both feet are flat on the floor. The movement resembles a march, with the emphasis on the downward action of the foot. Maintain an upright stance as the foot presses down.

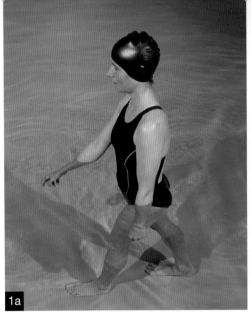

1a

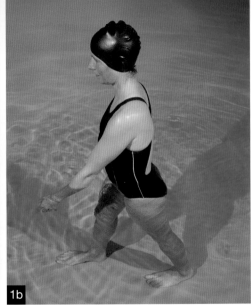

1b

- Pause for 3–4 seconds, and become aware of your balance and the relationship between your head, neck and back before taking a second step.
- Alternate the arms and legs, ensuring that the left leg moves forward and down as the right arm extends to counterbalance it (1a).
- Once you are comfortable with the timing, eliminate the pause and move continually (1b). You can also explore variations in pace, and explore deeper water. Walking more slowly encourages you to focus on balance and utilizes postural muscles. Speed and depth increase resistance, requiring more energy expenditure and resulting in more of a fitness workout.

Remember *Lead with the legs and let the arms follow; take small steps leading with the toe; place the heel down first. Keep the heel of the back foot down (feel the hamstring and calf muscles lengthen) until the other foot is fully in contact with the floor. This is essential in maintaining your sense of balance and forward direction. More effort is required to move in deeper water.*

Avoid *Don't walk too quickly, move the arm and leg on the same side together, fix the arms by the sides, cross the mid-line with arms or legs, look down or pull the head back, or overextend the arms by pushing them too far forward.*

2. Retro walking

Unless you work as a tour guide or a Shaw Method swimming teacher, you are unlikely to spend much time walking backwards, or retro walking. Research has shown that it is a valuable form of exercise, which is becoming increasingly popular with physiotherapists as a part of rehabilitation programmes. Retro walking is not simply the mirror image of forward walking; it calls for an increased range of motion in the knee joint and a similar reduction of movement in the hip. Walking backwards also requires more control of the trunk muscles, stretches the hamstrings and releases the hip flexors.

- Apart from aiding muscle balance and strengthening opposing muscles, retro walking in water has an additional benefit: it helps cultivate a greater awareness of the connection between the movement of the legs and the lower back. This skill is also essential when guiding or directing a partner, for example in the glide.
- From a standing position, lower the body by releasing the knees until the shoulders are at water level. Allow the arms to float in front of you with the palms upwards (2a).
- Gently press your lower back against the water and smoothly slide your feet over the floor (2b).

Remember *Connect with the floor, lead with the heels, release the lower back and widen across the shoulders.*

Avoid *Do not overbalance by leaning back with the upper back; do not lift the feet off the floor or move the head from side to side.*

3. The bellows

Moving sideways, unless you are trying to squeeze through a narrow space, is quite unfamiliar. Because of the reduction in frontal resistance, sideways movement through water is both easier as you experience the benefits of streamlining and harder as it is more difficult to balance. Sideways movement is particularly important in front and back crawl, where the aim is to minimize drag and maximize reach.

This practice familiarizes you with being on your side and teaches you how to incorporate a

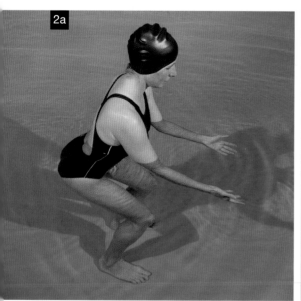

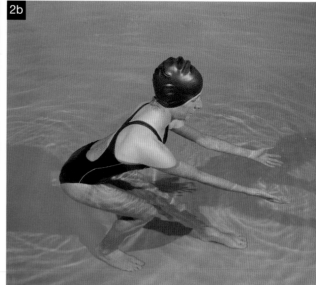

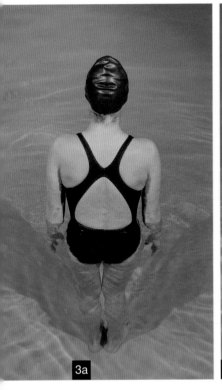

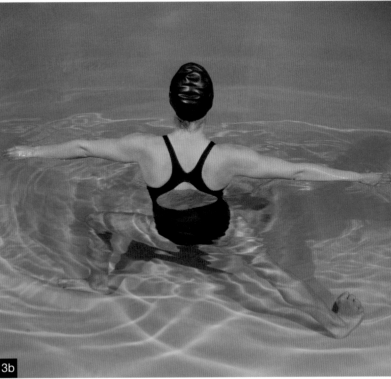

3a

3b

regulated breathing pattern as you widen with the effect of buoyancy, and lengthen in response to the water's resistance.

- Standing at full height, turn the body sideways with feet together, hands resting by your sides, and head centred. If the right side is leading, the eyes should look directly to the left throughout (3a).
- Elevate the left leg and step sideways, opening the arms to horizontal just above the surface of the water (3b). As the arms open, allow air to enter through the mouth.
- Draw the right leg towards the left and actively press the arms down until you are in

the original opening stance. As you press down, breathe out and think about lengthening along the spine (3a).

Remember *Allow the effects of buoyancy to assist the elevation of the arms and the process of breathing in. Pressing against the water provides the stimulus to breathe out. Like a pair of bellows, inflate as you open the arms and deflate as you close them.*

Avoid *Do not actively lift the arms, lean forward as the arms close, or twist the neck to look in the direction that you are travelling in.*

4. The lunge

This practice, which is performed by the wall of the pool, cultivates good alignment, giving you the opportunity to free the neck and feel how the arm extension originates from the back. It allows you to work on balance and stability in water whilst still being grounded through contact with the floor and walls of the pool. It is also a useful practice for making a smooth transition from standing upright to lying face down.

- Stand in the water, about a metre (3ft) away from the side of the pool.
- Place your right foot forward and gently release the knee; if possible keep the left heel on the floor – the effects of buoyancy make it more difficult to keep the heel down, which further encourages lengthening of the hamstrings.

- Maintain the head-neck-back relationship and extend both arms to the wall as the body tilts forward (hands are angled down with fingers below the wrists, wrists below elbows, elbows below shoulders and the head is in continuation of the spine).
- Generate an even pressure against the wall as you send the back backwards. Remain in this position for the count of ten (4a).
- Alternate the feet and notice if there are any differences between the left and right sides.

Remember *If possible, keep the heel flat on the floor to help lengthen the hamstrings and improve the relationship between the legs. The arms connect to the back; as they reach forward, the lower back is directed backwards.* **Avoid** *Do not pull the head back, bury the head, bend the elbows or arch the back.*

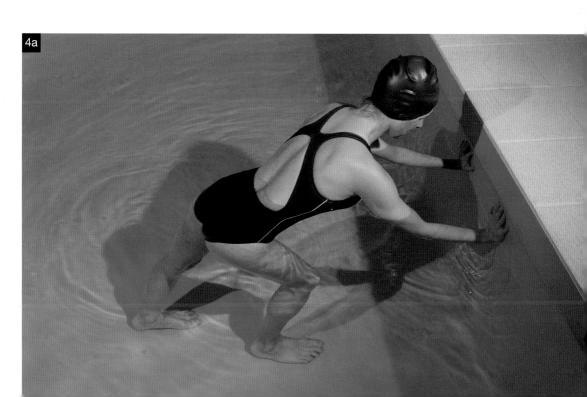

4a

* For a more difficult version of the practice, do it without the support of the wall, as it is harder to maintain balance and more of a challenge for the postural muscles.

5. Facing the water

Most people find the water a little cold when they first enter a pool, and it normally takes a minute or two to acclimatize. Wetting the face is a gentle way to approach facial immersion, teaching you to counteract the automatic tendency to tense up when water makes contact with the face. This practice can be very soothing, releasing tension in the jaw and neck.

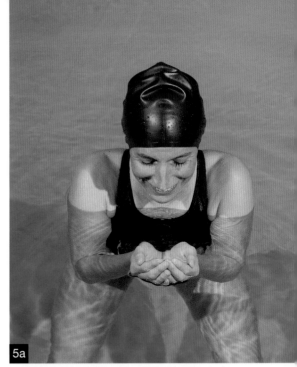

5a

- Without goggles (unless you are wearing contact lenses) cup both hands and collect water in your palms (5a).
- Softly close your eyes and slowly bring the water towards your forehead (5b). Explore your automatic reaction – is it to screw up your face, hold your breath or pull your head back as the water approaches?
- Work on inhibiting these automatic reactions and consciously soften your face as the water makes contact.
- Release tension in the jaw as you gently drag your hands down the face and over the eyelids, while slowly breathing out and saying 'Aah'. This often produces a very soothing sensation, which can be very helpful in releasing tension headaches.

Remember *Perform this action as slowly as possible; soften your chest and stomach as well as the face.*

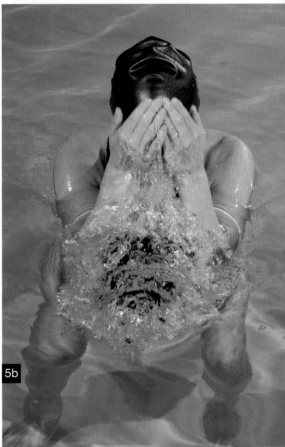

5b

Avoid Do not hold your breath, pull the head back, or tense the facial muscles.

6. Lunging with the face submerged

The next stage is to combine placing the face in the water with the lunge practice. To do this, it is preferable to wear goggles, open the eyes and look down at the floor. This can be performed with and without contact with the side of the pool, or with a partner supporting your wrists. It familiarizes you with the sensation of breathing out into water while having your feet firmly on the floor. As was discussed earlier, it is important to passively inhale prior to putting the face in the water, and to exhale gently into the water.

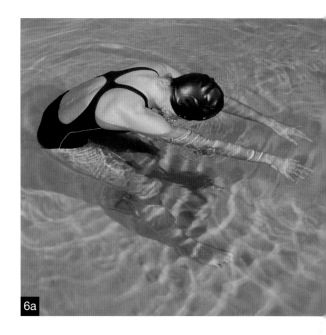

6a

- Stand in water no deeper than chest-level, facing the side of the pool and about a metre (3ft) away from it. Maintain this position for a few seconds, breathing in a relaxed and continuous manner, until you feel stable and balanced.
- With arms extended think about maintaining the length of your neck and back. With your right foot forward lower yourself down and place the face in the water. Gently start to exhale, saying 'Aah'.
- Continue to exhale as you lean into the water, with your weight shifting to the hands and front leg, until the mouth and nose are fully submerged. Gently exhale for around five seconds (6a).
- Before running low on breath, step forward with the left leg as you press down with the arms to raise the head and torso out of the

water. Maintain this upright stance for the count of five and then step back and repeat the practice, leading with the left leg. Wait until the water dribbles out of your mouth and nose before allowing the in-breath.

Remember Lengthen along the spine as you move between the vertical and horizontal plane. Those less familiar with putting their faces in the water may find it easier to do this practice with both feet parallel, bending at the knees, and only moving on to the one-foot-forward version when they feel confident and stable.

Avoid Don't take a large step, shorten the neck, or gasp or swallow air just before the face enters the water. Don't pull the head back, lift the arms up or arch the back.

7(i). The glide

A lack of poise and symmetry when swimming is often the result of not having spent sufficient time learning to be still in the water. Learning to glide and regain the feet in a balanced manner can have a very positive effect on one's overall sense of control in the water.

The glide is the ultimate opportunity to experience the tangible benefits of 'non-doing'. It calls for the capacity to trust the water as well as to lengthen and widen. When this is achieved, the glide brings a powerful sense of ease and liberation. Novices and competent swimmers alike often attempt to hold themselves up, instead of allowing the whole body to be supported by the water. This is often due to the misconception that if they do nothing they will sink. However, for most of us, when the water supports the head it actually takes more effort to sink than it does to float.

The glide is also an excellent way to really grasp the core Alexander Technique principle of leading with the head. When the whole body rests quietly just below the surface, the water gives us direct and accurate feedback on the quality of the relationship of the head, neck and back. If, for example, the head is orientated slightly off-centre, it will be very difficult to maintain a straight course.

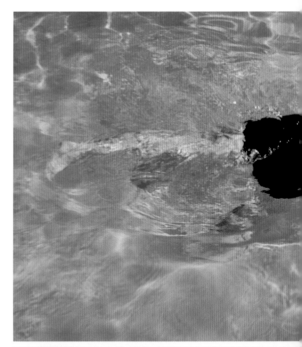

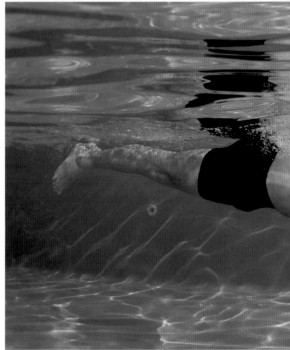

● Face the length or width of the pool and start as in the previous practice. This time, when you feel your weight transferring to the front foot, lean forward and start to exhale. Lean into the water as the head leads the movement into the horizontal plane (7[i]a).

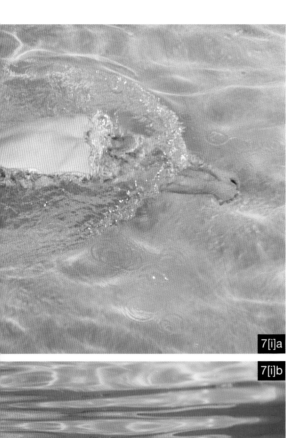

7[i]a

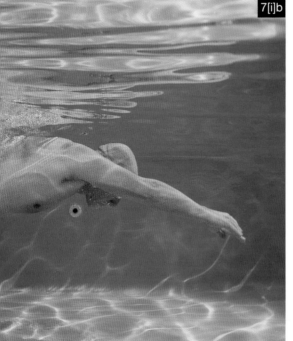

7[i]b

- Gently drift forward. Keep the arms relaxed, extended forward and angled slightly downward in order to maintain stability and prevent arching.
- Lengthen and widen the back while continuing to exhale gently.
- Keep the legs straight and together without locking the knees or lifting the hips (7[i]b).
- Maintain the glide for 5–6 seconds before starting to regain the feet (see 7ii).

Remember *Think of your head as a rudder, with the crown leading while the arms act as stabilizers. Trust the water to support you, and move at a slow steady pace, freeing the neck and releasing tension. Consciously relax the hands, which will promote a sense of letting go throughout the rest of the body.*

Avoid *Do not push off from the floor, snatch a breath just before the face enters the water, pull the head back at any point, hold the breath or exhale forcefully.*

7(ii). Finding the feet

The way in which most people automatically try to regain their feet from the glide is to pull the head back. (This is very similar to the way in which many stand from sitting.) The Shaw Method for finding the feet is a combination of tucking up the body as if to prepare to somersault, followed by a skipping action.

- Bow the head forward and down, flex the ankles and make your toes point to the floor by bending the knees and bringing the feet forward, curling up into a foetal position

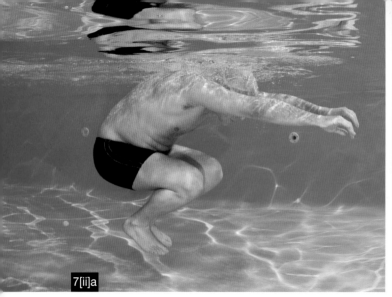
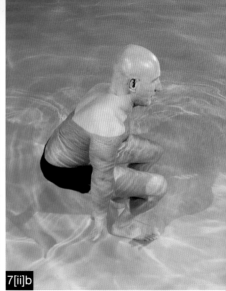

7[ii]a

7[ii]b

whilst maintaining the length and direction of the arms (7[ii]a).

- Gradually swing the arms towards the hips, tuck the pelvis under using the abdominals and muscles of the lower back. Begin to uncurl your spine and roll the head up so that the eyes look straight ahead.
- Land in a balanced manner with the feet parallel and firmly planted on the floor (7[ii]b). Extend to full height with the head centred.

Remember *Finding the feet from the glide is about getting down, not getting up – as long as you intend to get up it is very hard to inhibit the tendency to pull the head back. Enjoy the sense of curling and uncurling, and continue to breathe out as your face leaves the water.*
Avoid *Do not pull the head back or keep it pressed down as the arms sweep back. Do not pull the arms back before the tuck, as this will force the legs back up. Do not land on one foot.*

* For a more difficult version of the practice, do it with your arms by your sides, as it is harder to maintain balance and provides more of a challenge for the abdominal muscles.

8. Floating on the back

The ability to float on your back varies greatly from person to person. By learning to relax and extend the arms, many confirmed sinkers are surprised to find they can actually float. Attitudes to floating on the back also vary greatly: some people feel out of control while others feel more comfortable on their back than on their front. This practice will help less buoyant people float, and help 'extreme floaters' to regain their feet with ease.

- Prepare to float on your back.
- Without turning the head, release the knees and gradually lower the body into a crouch.
- Turn the palms upwards and gradually extend the arms to the side as you lean backwards (8a). Once both arms are

extended, take one foot and then the other off the floor and float on to your back. Continue to sweep the arms until they are fully extended behind the head, resembling the glide described previously (8b).

- To regain your feet, first tuck in the chin, then bend the ankles and knees (8c), and then finally sweep the arms round until they reach the surface with palms facing up (8d).

Remember *Free the neck to allow the weight of the head to be supported by the water. Release the shoulders as the arms move backwards and attempt to keep the arms submerged, with palms upward, throughout. When standing, tuck before using the arms – the face may get a little wet at first, but with practice you will be able to avoid this.*
Avoid *Do not throw the head backwards or lift it as you take off. Do not arch the back, lift the head or tilt it back in the glide. Do not stiffen the neck when regaining the feet.*

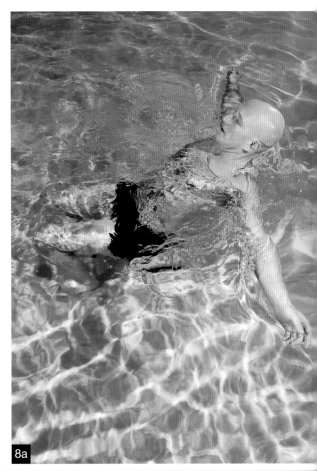

8a

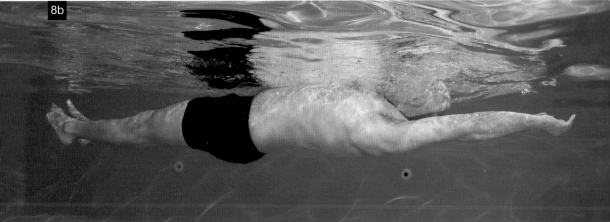

8b

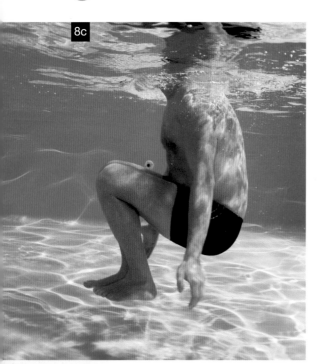

8c

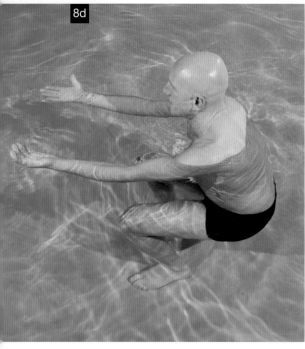

8d

9. Rotation

The ability to rotate provides a solid foundation for developing both the front and back crawl. This practice connects floating on the back with gliding on the front, utilizing a hip rotation to achieve the transition. It teaches breath control as you move from air to water, and reinforces the principle of leading with the head.

- Float on your back with your arms by your sides. If you tend to sink, perform a gentle, leg action to keep the feet up, but do not use them for propulsion.
- Allow the water to support the weight of the head and breathe gently. Aim to maintain this position for ten seconds (9a).
- Without moving the rest of the body, start looking towards your left shoulder.
- Allow the shoulder and then the hip to follow the movement of the head (9b) until you are face down and flat in the water, with your arms still by your sides.
- Breathe out in the transition between air and water. Remain floating, with your arms by your sides, for five seconds. Then tuck to regain your feet.
- Perform this movement again, looking towards the right shoulder. Most people have a preferred side.

Remember This movement feels like rolling a log: ensure that shoulders and hips remain loose to facilitate the movement. If you are uncomfortable regaining your feet with your arms by your sides, feel free to extend them.

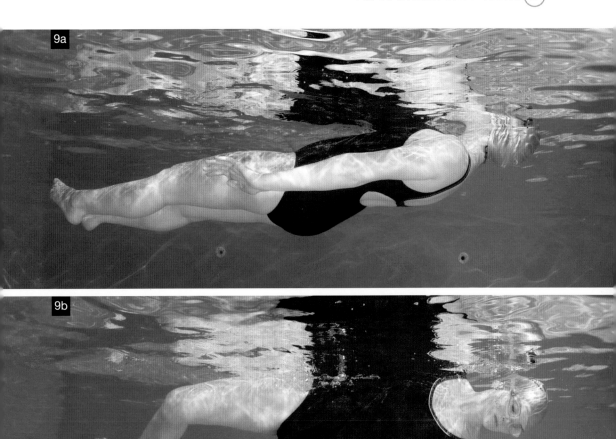

9a

9b

Avoid *Do not lead the rotation with any body part other than the head. Do not close the eyes and/or hold your breath as your face becomes immersed. Do not pull the head back when regaining the feet.*

10. The wave

All the previous practices are performed on either a vertical or horizontal plane; this practice allows you to explore movement between these planes. It also gives you the opportunity to experiment with different depths and the upthrust of the water, which is important in both

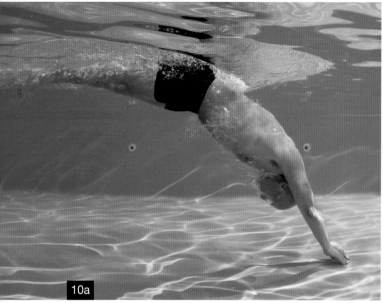

10a

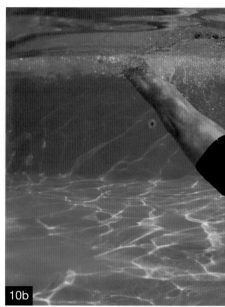

10b

the breaststroke and butterfly strokes.

The wave is a great confidence-building practice, which also mobilizes the spine. Many people initially find it challenging, but then it becomes fun and exhilarating. The key is to focus on directing the body forward and not simply up and down.

● Step forward into a regular glide and gently start to exhale. Maintain this position for a few seconds until you feel stable.
● Raise the eyes to look straight ahead, tilting the head slightly backward. Keep the arms extended and release the knees.
● Actively press the head, neck and shoulders down, hollow the chest and allow the head to lead the rest of the body in a forward and slightly downward direction (10a). Straighten the legs with some force, contract the

abdominals to lift the hips, which then follow the movement of the upper body towards the floor (10b).
● Keeping the arms extended, gradually look upwards towards the surface. Open the chest and allow the body to glide forward and up towards the surface.
● When your eyes see the surface of the water from below, tuck in the head and regain your feet (10c).

Remember *The downward movement is active and the upward is passive. Flow through the movement (little effort is required) and allow the hips and lower back to move in a wave-like action. As you descend, exhale through the nose to avoid the unpleasant sensation of water flooding the sinuses.*
Avoid *Do not shorten the arms to pull the body*

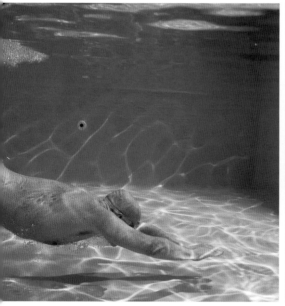

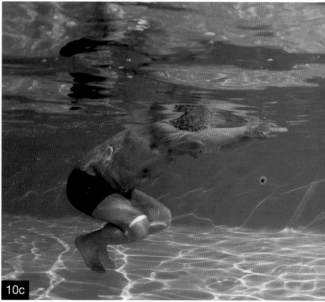

10c

down, or breathe out too forcefully as this will
make it harder to float back up. Do not pull the
head back too far as you come up.

Swimming different strokes

To appreciate the wider health benefits of
swimming, it is important to swim a combination
of strokes. Apart from working different parts of
the body, each stroke engages the brain in
different ways and produces differing
sensations. Although some people clearly have
an affinity or preference for a certain stroke, no
stroke is intrinsically more difficult than another.
Unless there is a medical reason for avoiding a
stroke (such as a hip replacement, which
makes the breaststroke leg action unsafe), we
all have the capacity to perform each stroke in
a relaxed and confident way. Many people with
chronic back conditions believe that they must

avoid the breaststroke and butterfly. In my
experience, swimming these strokes with the
Shaw Method can do more to relieve back pain
than back or front crawl. If you are in doubt, talk
to a health professional about your concerns.

CHECKPOINTS
- Are there other physical activities that
  you approach in an unthinking way?
- What are the factors that affect your
  ability to float?
- Are you aware of day-to-day situations
  in which you pull your head back?
- Can you think of circumstances when it
  is appropriate to hold your breath?

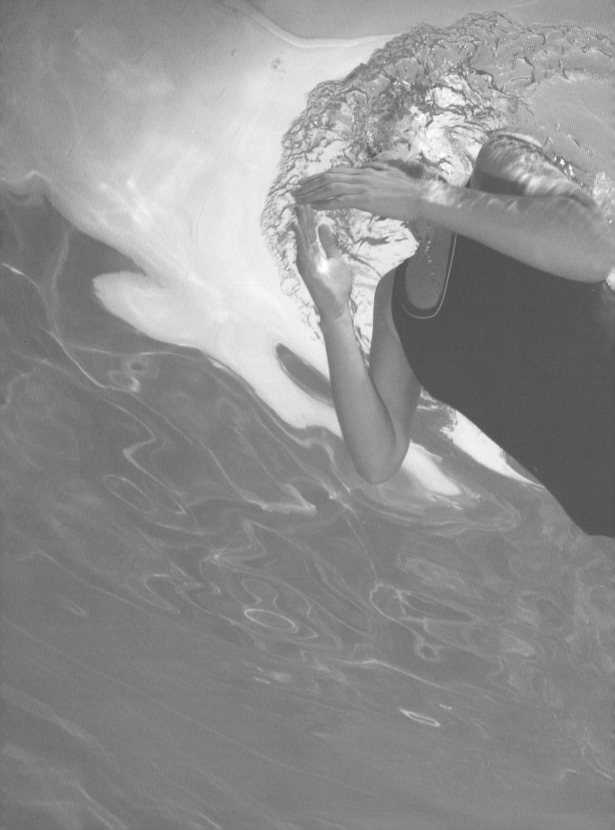

BREASTSTROKE
WITH EASE

'The gentle undulation and glide helps to unwind the body and clear the mind.'

Deborah Stevens, registered Shaw Method teacher

Breaststroke has existed since prehistoric times. Stone Age paintings featuring a similar stroke were found in the 'cave of swimmers' near Wadi Sora in Egypt. It was the only stroke permitted during the great plague in the Middle Ages, because swimmers could keep their faces out of the water and therefore would not, it was believed, spread the epidemic.

Breaststroke was also the preferred stroke in Victorian Britain, where an overarm action was deemed inelegant and unsuitable for ladies and gentlemen. It was the original competitive stroke and was popularized by Captain Webb who, in 1875, became the first man to swim the English Channel.

In the UK and many other parts of the world, breaststroke remains the most popular stroke today. Its relative stability, with the arms and legs working in tandem, makes it accessible to swimmers of all levels. For many, its appeal is the long glide where the arms and legs are still as the swimmer advances; others appreciate that it strengthens and tones their legs, whilst some choose it as the best means of keeping their hair dry!

Breaststroke is easy to swim but hard to swim well; despite its popularity few are able to perform the stroke in a way that promotes good overall 'use'. Many swim with their heads held up out of the water, placing great pressure on the spine. Even if people swim with their face in the water, they rarely have an effective arm and leg action or good timing.

Furthermore, because most have swum this stroke regularly since childhood, detrimental habits have become so strongly ingrained that the prospect of change is more challenging than with a less familiar stroke.

There is little point in tinkering with individual elements of the stroke: the best recipe for success is to recraft it from scratch. The following three breaststroke lessons take you through a series of practices covering the core elements of the stroke. Only when you have firmly established an effective arm and leg action are you ready to progress to the more complex process of coordinating the stroke and integrating the breath.

Shaw Method key features

Orientation Low, both in the glide, where the neck is fully extended with the eyes looking straight down, and in the breathing position, where the chin rests near the surface.

Arm action In the initial glide position, the arms are directed slightly downward. Little effort is expended in the opening phase as the upper back widens; in the propulsive movement, the focus is on holding the water to draw the torso forward and up, as opposed to pulling the arms back.

Leg action We stress the importance of the non-propulsive element of the leg action, where the legs release before actively pushing back. We advocate a wide, wedge-like action as opposed to the narrower, more common whip kick, because it promotes hip mobility and reduces the risk of knee injury.

Rhythm In the competitive model, where the objective is to move into the propulsive actions as quickly as possible, a long glide is perceived as a waste of time. Breaststroke according to the Shaw Method is a series of glides punctuated by active movements. The glide is at the heart of the stroke, giving the swimmer more time to release the breath and lengthen and widen the back.

Benefits

Breaststroke can improve the mobility of many joints including the hips, shoulders, ankles, wrists and spine. As a leg-dominant stroke, the breaststroke strengthens and tones the quadriceps at the front of the legs and the hamstrings at the back. This is also the reason why breaststroke can be an effective way of improving aerobic fitness, as despite being the slowest stroke, it burns the most calories. Many find the long glide, where the swimmer gently exhales, particularly calming and meditative. Because of the inherent stability of the stroke, it is often a comfortable way to begin to explore the transition between air and water.

Risks and common mistakes

Alignment

1. The common practices of craning the neck and snatching it out of the water to breathe puts strain on the spine and can create a whiplash-type injury.
2. Permanently holding the head high, both in the glide and the breathing phases, increases drag/resistance as well stiffening the neck and creating a hump. For every inch the head is lifted, the hips sink two inches.
3. In competitive breaststroke, coaches encourage swimmers to hunch their shoulders in order to maximize the streamlining of the body, usually resulting in poor posture and shallow breathing.

Timing

1. Many swimmers have difficulty coordinating this stroke, and the arm and leg actions are often executed simultaneously. This not only reduces the propulsive effects of the limbs, but produces a concertina-like effect which strains the back.
2. Hurriedly pulling the heels towards the seat can also injure the lower back.
3. A short glide does not provide sufficient time to exhale comfortably, which can give rise to an erratic breathing pattern and even to hyperventilation.

Propulsion

1. If you apply too much effort to open the arms, and open them too wide, it not only increases drag but can also significantly reduce the effectiveness of the arm action.
2. Most knee injuries are related to the use of the whip kick (see glossary). 'Breaststroker's knee' is the result of repeated stress on the medial collateral ligament.
3. A lack of awareness or inflexibility in either hip hinders the ability to produce a symmetrical leg action. The resulting 'screw kick' not only produces an uneven thrust and twist of the spine, but once established it is very difficult to unlearn.

LESSON 1: ARM ACTION

The sculling arm action (see glossary) in breaststroke promotes flexibility of the wrist, elbow and shoulder joints. It is an ideal antidote to the sustained arm position of many keyboard users, which often results in repetitive strain injury (RSI). Similar fluid arm movements are also integral to martial arts.

The aim of this lesson is to develop a smooth, rhythmical and effective arm action. Unlike front crawl and backstroke, where the upper body is dominant, breaststroke is leg-dominant and the main purpose of the arms is to elevate the torso to facilitate inhalation. This action, during which the hands remain submerged, has four phases: extension, opening out, the pull–lift phase, and recovery. The key to achieving an effective arm action is to apply minimal effort during the non-propulsive phases and the appropriate amount of drive during the propulsive phase.

This lesson takes you through a series of practices that cover the component parts of the arm action, showing you how to time and coordinate them correctly. To avoid stressing the neck and back, the face remains in the water during horizontal practices. Remember: as breaststroke is a leg-dominant stroke, it is unnecessary to apply a lot of effort with the arms.

1. Scooping

This practice can be performed in the pool or on dry land. The aim is to coordinate the various phases of the arm action without hunching the shoulders or narrowing the back. As a stationary practice, it encourages you to

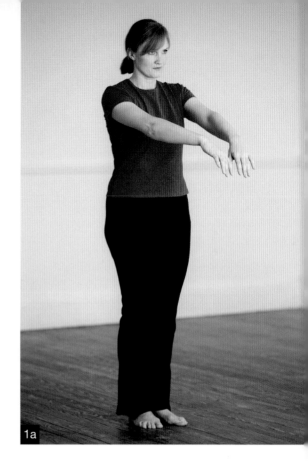
1a

focus on the quality of movement without the distraction of achieving forward motion.

- Start in the opening stance; maintain this position for a few seconds to achieve balance and stability.
- Extend the arms forward and slightly down, elbows below shoulders, wrists below elbows, fingers below wrists, hands side by side, palms down (1a). The head-neck-back should be well aligned with the eyes looking at the hands; the breathing relaxed and continuous throughout.
- Count to three, then gently rotate your palms outward and begin to open your arms (1b),

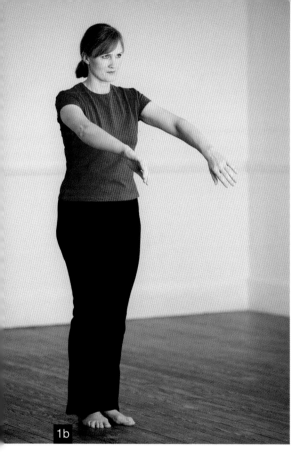

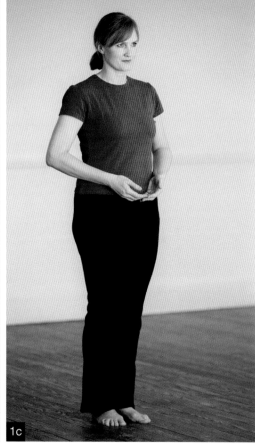

1b

1c

starting the movement across the back, until they arrive just beyond shoulder width by the count of five. Maintain the length of the arms and the depth of the hands.

- On the count of six, rotate the wrists so that the palms are facing inwards and actively scoop the hands in towards the stomach. By the count of seven, the hands should have formed a loose, cupping position just below the ribs (1c).
- On the count of eight, direct the hands forward and down, until the arms are fully lengthened without locking elbows, with the palms facing down and the hands together (1a). With the eyes looking straight ahead,

maintain a balanced, lengthened position for two beats. Repeat the sequence.

Remember *Stand tall, keeping the neck long and the eyes looking straight ahead. Perform the opening phases with minimal effort. Think about the lower back staying back and relax the hands as the arms move forward.*

Avoid *Do not lock the arms and angle them up in the initial extension and recovery phases. Do not collapse the chest as the arms open out. Do not hunch the shoulders or bring the elbows behind the torso in the scooping phase.*

2. Stepping

This practice, in addition to reinforcing the correct arm action, will develop your appreciation of the connection between arms and breathing pattern. Here the objective is to utilize the resistance of the water to pull the body forward, as opposed to sweeping the arms backwards. It requires you to synchronize the movement of the arms with a step – a good foundation to draw upon during the later stages of coordinating the arm and leg actions.

- Step forward with the right leg and simultaneously extend the arms forward and down as you start to exhale gently (2a).
- With your weight spread evenly on both feet, widen the back and open the arms, continuing to exhale slowly (2b).

- With a scooping arm action, bring the left foot forward in line with the other leg. Allow the air to come in through the mouth (2c).
- Breathe out as you step forward with the left foot and simultaneously extend your arms; both feet now share your weight equally.
- Repeat the sequence with the other foot leading, noticing any differences.

Remember *In the opening phase, maintain the length of the arms. Keep the head centred and the neck long throughout. Take your time – there is no need to hurry.*
Avoid *Do not step forward out of sequence, i.e. before the arms start their recovery. Do not sweep the arms back.*

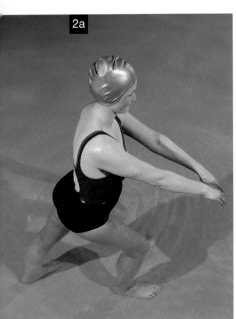
2a

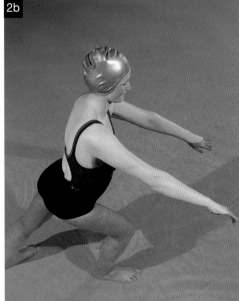
2b

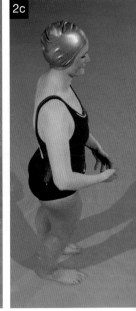
2c

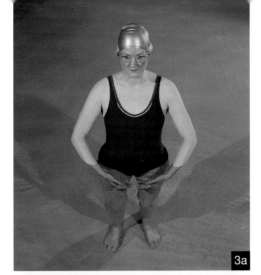

3a

3. Step and glide

In breaststroke, the glide is very much at the heart of the stroke and this practice reinforces its importance. For many people, the process of lengthening along the spine is easier to recognize when they are standing up than when they are face down in the water. Here the smooth transition between vertical and horizontal is a reminder to lengthen in the water.

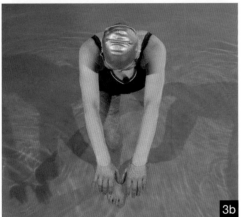

3b

- Start as in the previous practice and perform one complete cycle of the combined arm and stepping practice. Pause at the end of the sequence (3a).
- Begin to exhale as you shift your weight on to the right foot and with the head leading, angle the body down into a well-balanced glide with the eyes looking at the floor. Ensure that the front foot makes full contact with the floor and is carrying your body weight before launching off (3b).
- Maintain the glide for a few seconds as you allow the water to support you; lengthen and widen your back (3c).
- Tuck to regain the feet and then repeat the action with the left leg leading.

Remember *You may be surprised by how far you travel – the momentum gained by stepping into the glide is quite significant. Keep the hands soft throughout.*
Avoid *Do not stumble as a result of not putting the foot down firmly before taking off. Do not snatch a breath or pull the head back when going into the glide.*

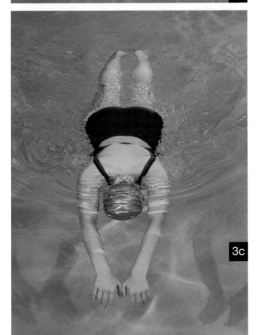

3c

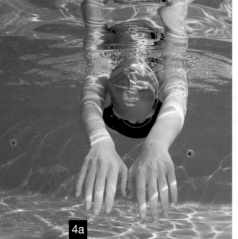

4a

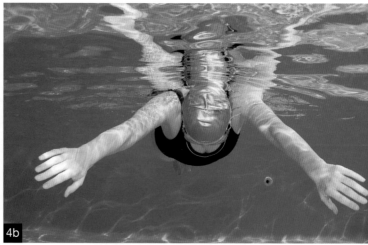

4b

4. Floating arms

The aim of this practice is to move from an extended glide into the opening-out phase whilst maintaining the length and direction of the arms. This action creates a stable base prior to the application of propulsive effort.

- Step forward into a well-balanced glide, with thumbs touching and palms face down. Maintain this position as you breathe out for three or four seconds (4a).
- Gently rotate your palms outwards and begin to float the arms apart so that they are a little wider than the width of your shoulders. Do not apply much effort: a good analogy here is to imagine lengthening a fine thread (4b).
- Maintain this position for a further 3–4 seconds before tucking to regain your feet. If you float well and have the ability to relax your breathing, you can repeat this practice two or three times before regaining your feet.

Remember *Imagine balancing on a narrow beam when the hands are together and on a wider beam when they are apart. Allow this widening movement to originate from the back.* **Avoid** *Do not raise the head, tense the arms or sweep them back.*

5. Arm action

This practice integrates the different arm movements on the horizontal plane and requires the ability to trickle breathe (see glossary). Without the distraction of the leg action, you can give the quality of this movement your full attention.

- Inhale lightly and launch into a stable glide; maintain for three seconds with a free neck and the eyes looking straight down. Breathe out gently (5a).
- Widen the back and slide the arms apart to just beyond shoulder width, palms and eyes down; continue to breathe out gently (5b).

- Scoop the hands and forearms down and towards each other (5c). The palms come together just in front of the chest (5d). Continue to exhale.
- Extend the arms forward and down, until they are fully lengthened with the palms facing down and hands together. Continue the exhalation in a stable glide for a further three seconds and regain the feet.
- Repeat the practice twice before regaining the feet. Be sure to breathe out gently.

Remember *Maintain the head-neck-back alignment with your face in the water throughout. If your feet sink, lower the head a little or paddle to keep them up.*

Avoid *Do not exhale explosively, as this reduces your ability to float. Do not pull the elbows behind the shoulders, as it narrows the upper back and encourages arching. Do not lock the arms or direct them upward in the recovery.*

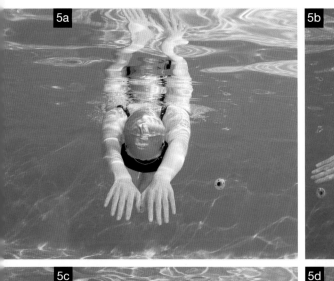

5a

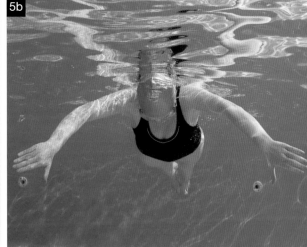

5b

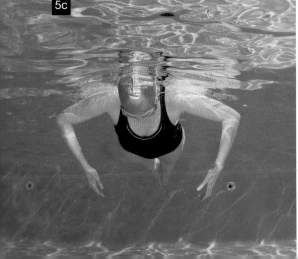

5c

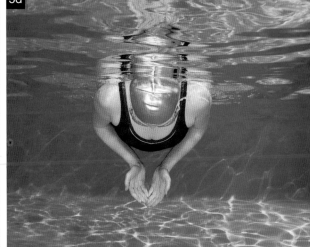

5d

LESSON 2: LEG ACTION

As people age, their range of motion, particularly of the hips, knees and ankles, tends to reduce and many develop arthritis from wear and tear. The inflexibility of these weight-bearing joints is often cited as a major reason for the increasing number of hip and knee replacements. Most do very little in their daily lives to promote suppleness in these areas and without targeted flexibility exercises, the abductor muscles around these joints inevitably seize up over time.

An efficient breaststroke leg action is a simple and effective way to maintain the health of the hip joint and promote overall leg flexibility.

In Japanese culture, the common practice of sitting on the floor requires significant hip abduction (movement away from the centre-line), which results in lower rates of arthritis in the lower limbs. It is no coincidence that the Japanese are particularly adept at breaststroke and their swimmers have had a great deal of success in this stroke.

The leg action provides most of the forward thrust in breaststroke, producing around 70 per cent of the overall propulsion. The symmetrical action of the legs resembles the movement of a swimming frog – hence the term 'frog kick'. In competitive swimming, a narrow, streamlined leg action known as the whip kick is favoured.

In the Shaw Method, a wider action, which places less stress on the knees, is preferred. This movement consists of two phases: the preparatory phase and the thrust phase.

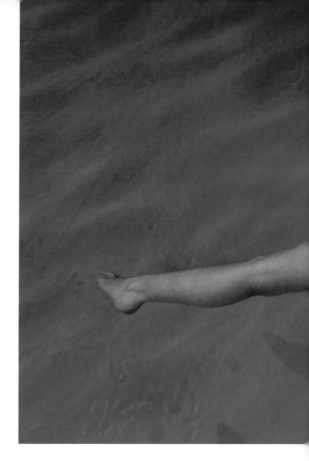

- **Preparatory** From the glide with the legs extended backward, the ankles are released to allow the feet to turn slightly outward. The heels are drawn gently towards the posterior as the thighs and knees are turned out.

- **Thrust** The legs are driven backwards and inwards to the glide position, gaining force and pace throughout the movement. Propulsion is gained through a combination of driving the legs back and drawing them together.

In an effective leg action, the feet change plane. They move from being close to the

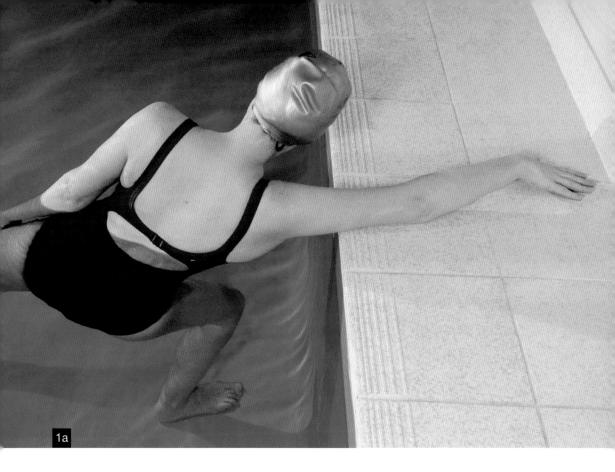

1a

surface of the water during the glide, to a few inches below the surface, and then back up in a wave-like motion.

In the following practices, the legs are isolated from the arms, enabling you to focus on this critical aspect of the stroke. Separating the arm and leg actions is also an effective means of breaking the unhelpful pattern of moving them simultaneously.

1. Leg extension

This practice promotes flexibility in the hip, thigh and groin areas, which is essential in an effective breaststroke leg action. It also highlights the importance of good alignment.

- Stand in shallow water, at right angles to the edge of the pool. Extend the right arm and rest it on the poolside; ensure that the right foot is firmly on the floor, facing forwards.
- Release the left arm so it rests by the left hip and rotate the torso to the left. Take the left foot off the floor and allow it to lengthen as it floats up (1a).
- Keep the right hand firmly in contact with the side as the left leg rises and extends. Point the toes in line with the leg.

Remember *Free the neck and head in continuation of the spine and allow the leg to lengthen out from the hip.*

Avoid *Do not lift the leg too high and arch the back, twist the back, push the head down, or twist the front foot so that the toes turn inward.*

2. Sumo stance

This practice familiarizes you with turning both feet out evenly and opening the hips into what is for most an unfamiliar, frog-like position. It promotes a symmetrical leg action – one of the hallmarks of an efficient breaststroke. It also addresses the importance of not arching the back as the knees bend.

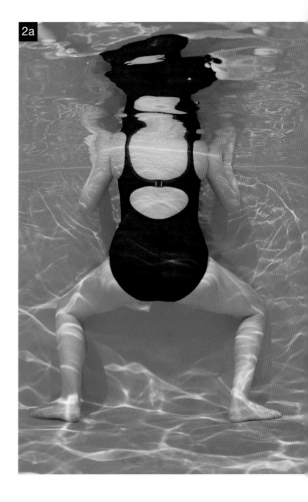

2a

- Think of releasing the neck and place the hands on the side of the pool. Stand facing the poolside, a little way away from it, in water no deeper than chest level. The knees should be hip-width apart, and the feet turned out slightly and away from the wall.
- Bend the knees and direct them outward as you lower yourself a few inches. The inner knees should make light contact with the wall.
- Gently press the knees into the wall. Notice a gentle stretch running along the inside of the thighs and hips (2a).
- Continue to exert gentle pressure for 10 seconds before standing up to full height and relaxing both legs. Repeat this practice at least three times.

Remember *Direct knees outward, keep heels in contact with the floor, ensure that the tailbone drops aways and the knees move in ine with the toes.*
Avoid *Do not hollow the back or twist the pelvis. Do not exert more pressure on one side*

or turn either foot inward. Do not let the head fall forward or pull it back.

3. Supported frog

Here, comfortably supported by the side of the pool, you can gently practice the full leg action with a clear view and without the distraction of trying to get anywhere. It clearly emphasizes the difference between the releasing and active phases of the leg action. This practice works particularly well in deck-level pools.

- Stand with your back against the corner of the pool. Place the elbows on the side of the pool and lift the legs to float just below the surface. Extend the legs and maintain this position for four beats (3a).
- Release the ankles and knees (so they drop a few inches), gently draw the feet into the frog position and breathe in. Pay attention to establishing and maintaining symmetry (3b).
- Push outward with the soles (3c), then turn the feet inwards and actively bring both legs towards each other; exhale gently (3a). Maintain the extension for four beats whilst continuing to breathe out gently.

Remember *Release the hips and stomach muscles in the first phase and contract them in the dynamic phase.*

Avoid *Do not snatch the legs in forcefully, as this will sabotage the propulsive phase.*

4. Frog with the face down

Here, the non-propulsive phase of the leg action is practiced separately. When you are on your front, it can be hard to avoid following the unhelpful pattern of the feet breaking the surface, but here you have an opportunity to correct this before putting any effort into the leg action, which can be injurious if the legs are too high in the water.

In full breaststroke, this phase corresponds to the opening and scooping of the arms and therefore needs to be slow enough to allow sufficient time to perform both arm movements.

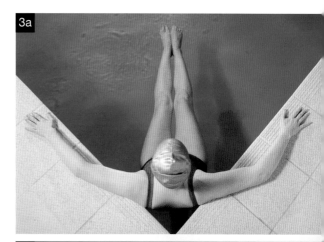

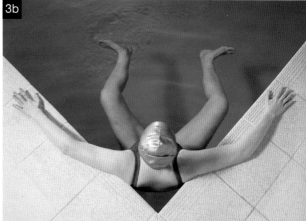

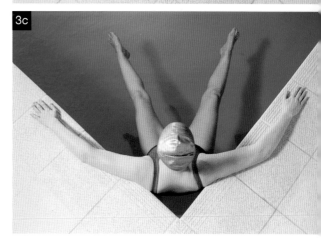

- Step forward, extend the arms and drift off into a glide with the feet together, arms directed forward and down, and eyes looking straight down. Maintain this glide for four beats.
- Turn the toes out, release the ankles and knees, and slowly draw the heels towards the posterior (4a).
- Maintain this position for four beats. Lengthen and draw both legs together without thrusting, then regain the feet.
- Repeat the frog with face down sequence until it is balanced, with both feet symmetrical.

Remember *Think about primary control, and opening the legs without effort. Keep both feet submerged at all times.*

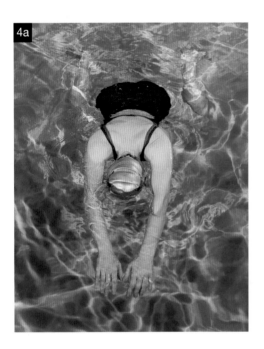

4a

Avoid *Do not lift the head or arch the back, pull the feet up with effort or bring them up to the posterior (this can strain the lower back).*

5. One leg at a time

This practice familiarizes you with the movement of the legs while you are on your front. By working a single leg, it is easier to tell if there are any differences between the left and right side. It is also a helpful way to work on the tempo of the leg action.

- Stand at 90° to the wall of the pool, in water no deeper than shoulder height.
- Place the left hand on the side of the pool, the left foot on the floor, and rotate the right hip outwards to allow the right foot to float behind with the toes pointed (5a).
- Release the right leg so it sinks a few inches and rotate the ankle joint to turn the foot out.
- Release the right knee and gently draw the foot towards your seat. Pause for a couple of seconds (5b).
- In a single continuous movement, actively thrust the right leg out until it is fully extended and then draw it back towards the centre.
- Repeat five times with the right leg and then change to the left, noting any differences.

Remember *Direct the knee and foot outwards as the head remains centred.*
Avoid *Do not shorten the neck, actively draw in the leg instead of releasing it, or turn the knee of the standing leg inward.*

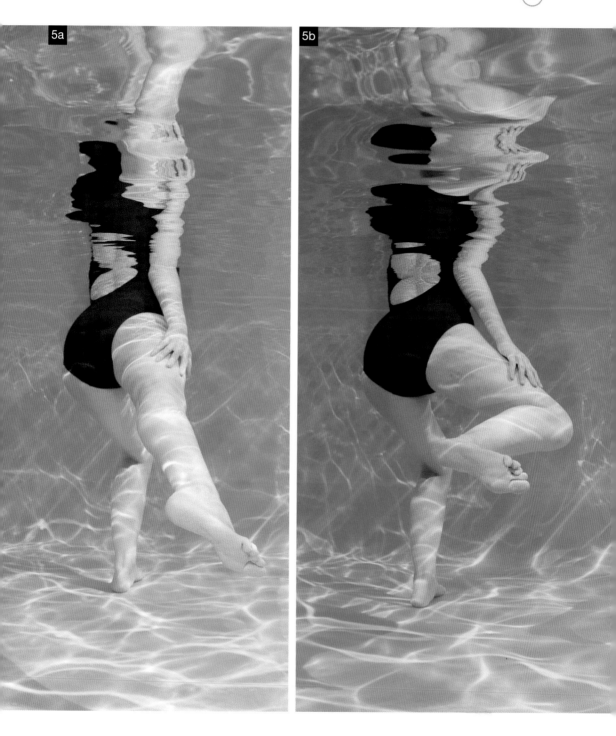

5a

5b

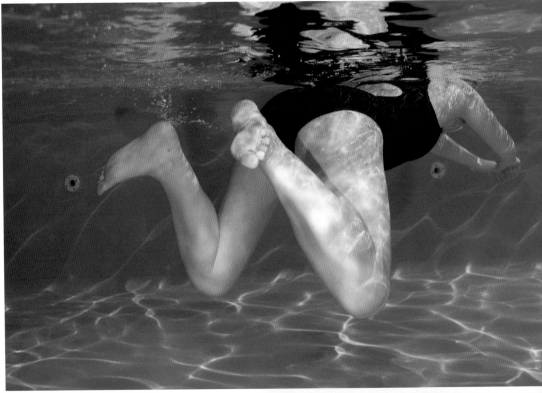

6. Complete leg action

In this practice, the arms do not move but their position is vital to the functioning of the legs. If they are placed too high, this will arch the back, making it harder to generate propulsive force (it is also potentially injurious). If you tend to move the arms and legs together, you may feel a compulsion to bend the arms when the legs start to move: this must be avoided.

- Launch into a glide, point the toes and extend the legs without locking the knees.
- Turn the feet out to allow the ankles, knees and hips to rotate outwards. Release the

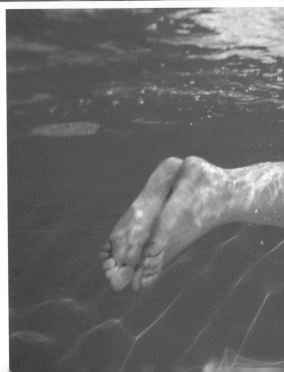

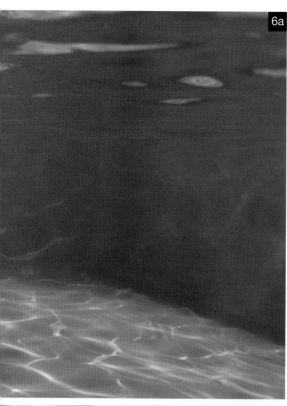

6a

ankles and knees, and draw the feet towards the seat as the hips widen (6a).

- Sequence: ankles, knees and then hips in one gentle, controlled movement. Maintain the second glide for four beats and then stand before repeating.
- Drive the feet back and out. As the knees straighten, turn and point the feet and draw the legs together into a glide (6b).

Remember *Observe how an effective kick allows the whole body to be directed dynamically forward in one horizontal plane, with your head leading.*

Avoid *Do not shorten the arms as the knees bend, make an uneven or screw kick, or pull the head back. If one ankle or hip is stiff, it may be difficult to achieve a symmetrical leg action, which will inevitably push the body off balance.*

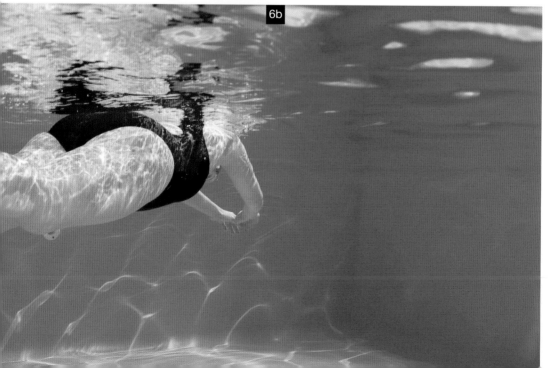

6b

LESSON 3: TIMING AND BREATHING

Timing

When working to establish the correct timing in breaststroke, it is useful to remember the function of the arms and legs. The primary purpose of the arms is to lift your body forward and up, and the role of the legs is to push you forward and down. So the objective, when combining arms and legs, is to release the legs as the arms perform their propulsive action, and to extend the arms when the legs thrust. Never open the arms until the legs are closed. The body is travelling at maximum velocity at the end of the leg action, so enjoy the glide.

Breathing

During the glide, a gradual exhalation through the mouth takes place underwater. The face is elevated to breathe, which is the combined result of a scooping arm action, which raises the upper body, and the release of the knees, which causes the hips to descend. A minimal movement of the head is all that is required to comfortably inhale through the mouth at the end of the pull–lift phase.

1. Chair practice

Before attempting to combine the arm and leg action in the water, it is helpful to practise on dry land. Standing upright, you can work for a sustained period on coordination, timing and rhythm without having to stop to take a breath.

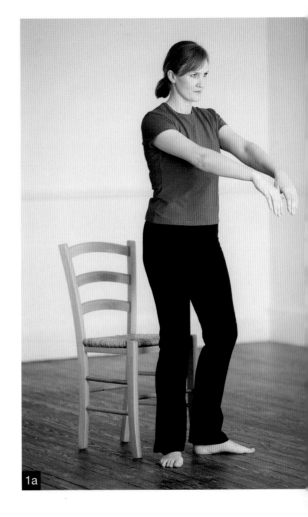

1a

- Stand in front of a chair with the arms extended, feet spread around hip-width apart and turned out, and legs extended to the count of 1, 2, 3, 4 (1a).
- Open the arms gently and broaden across the back (count 5, 6) (1b).
- Release the wrists and scoop the hands in towards the stomach. Bend the elbows (7) and then the knees (8) to sit at the edge of the chair (1c).
- Push up with the legs (9) and extend the arms forward (10), with the eyes looking straight

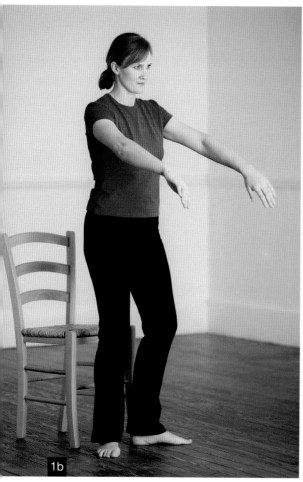

1b

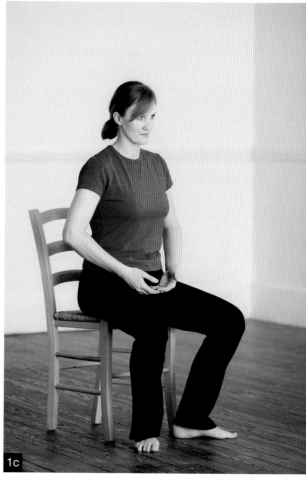

1c

ahead (1a). Repeat this until the timing feels comfortable, then remove the chair and perform the action without support. This practice also works well standing in water.

Remember *Arms lead the first part of the stroke and the legs lead the second. Keep the heels in contact with the floor throughout.*
Avoid *Do not lean forwards, sway backwards, bend the knees before the arms have started*

their scoop, or finish the arm extension before the legs start to straighten.

2. Glide – arms and legs
Here you return to the previous lessons to consolidate your learning. Since it has been a while since you worked on the glide and arm actions, it is a good idea to re-familiarize yourself with them before attempting to combine the two.

- Step into the glide with the eyes looking down at the floor and the crown of the head leading. Maintain the glide for 4–5 seconds before regaining the feet.
- Perform one complete sequence of arm movements with the face in the water and legs together. Regain the feet.
- Perform one complete sequence of leg actions with the arms extended and regain the feet.
- Return to the glide and repeat the sequence of glide, stand; arms, stand; legs, stand at least three times.

Remember *Think about the quality and tempo of each separate action in isolation, breathing out gently when the face is submerged.*
Avoid *Do not shorten the neck, perform more than one leg or arm action each time, or move the legs when working on the arms and vice versa.*

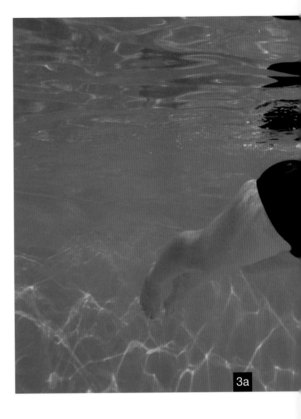

3a

3. Arm with legs

Having revised the separate elements, you are now ready to integrate them. Here it is useful to remind yourself that the breaststroke is a leg-dominant stroke, and to avoid putting too much effort into the arm action. If you are dissatisfied with any part of the action, ignore the temptation to repeat it before regaining your feet – it is far better to stand up and start the movement again.

- Breathe in gently, step forward and drift into a glide. Breathe out lightly and maintain this position, with hands together and palms facing down, for a count of 1, 2, 3, 4 (3a).

- Gently rotate the hands outwards and open them to shoulder-width apart. Maintain your head position, with the eyes looking straight down, and continue to exhale (5, 6) (3b).
- Relax the wrists and scoop towards the torso. Turn the feet out and draw the heels effortlessly towards the seat (7, 8) (3c).
- Extend the feet out and away, pushing the water with the whole of the feet. Close the legs (9) and lengthen the arms forward and down into the water (10) (3d).

Remember *Perform a pulling action with the arms, followed by a push from the legs. It is easier to coordinate the two if you move slowly.*

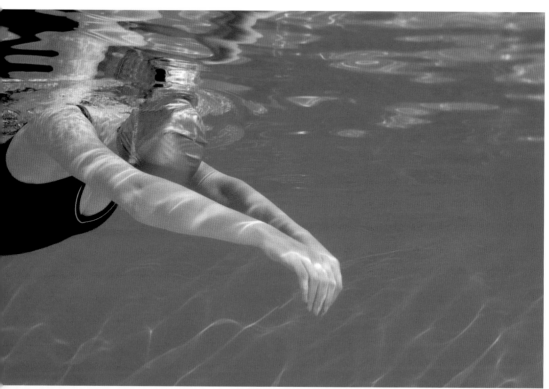

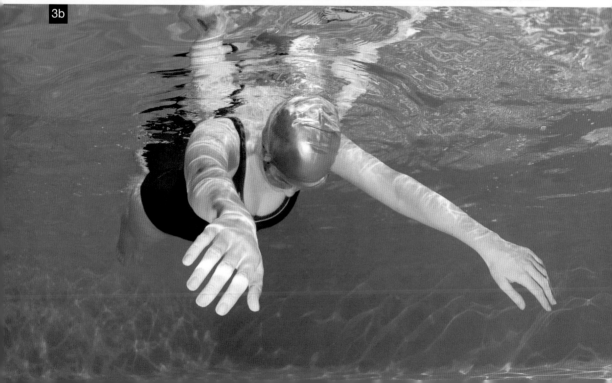

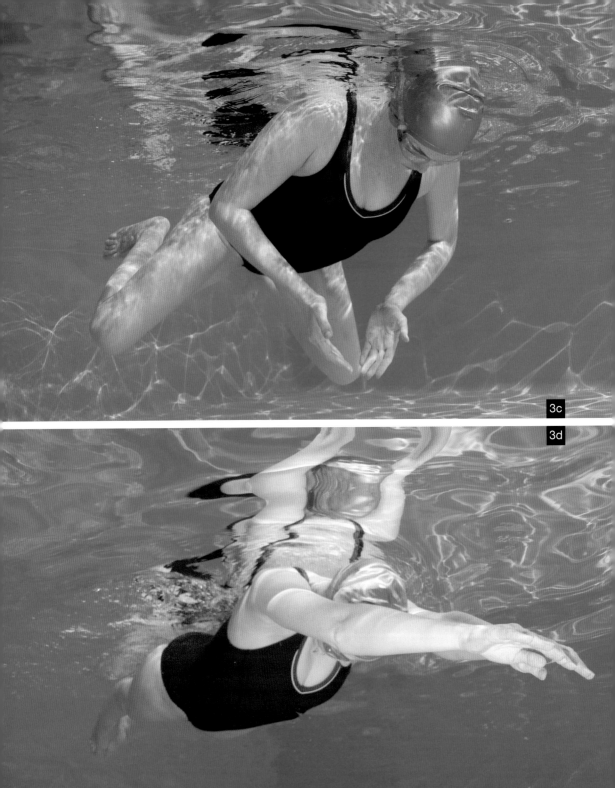

3c

3d

Avoid Do not execute arm and leg actions at the same time, apply too much effort with the arms or legs, or lift the head to inhale.

4. Rolling the head

The Alexander Technique emphasizes the importance of a free neck and the dangers of forcefully pulling the head back. This is sometimes misinterpreted as meaning that there is a correct position in which to hold the head. A free neck allows you to move the head from side to side and up and down, not to hold it in a fixed position. The ability to nod freely is vital in achieving an effective breathing position in breaststroke. Locate your so-called 'nodding' joint before you do this practice. Place the tips of your fore-fingers just beneath your ears and gently nod your head, notice that your fingers do not move.

- Standing with feet together and arms by your sides, tilt forward and inhale lightly (4a).
- Look down at floor, lengthening the neck and gently breath out to the count of 1, 2, 3.
- Roll the head so that the eyes are raised, continuing to exhale (count 4, 5) (4b).
- Raise the chin in line with the shoulders and allow air to come in through the mouth (6, 7).
- Bow the head, allowing the forehead to lead the movement (8, 9) and begin to exhale (4a). Repeat this series of movements a number of times until the nodding joint feels free.
- It is beneficial to perform this practice on dry land first, and then in the pool with the water level at shoulder height, and the face moving in and out of the water.

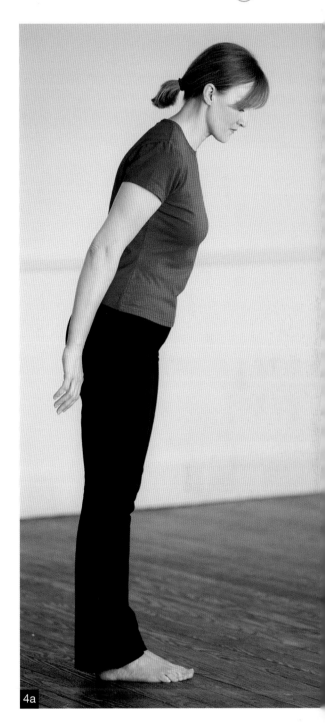

4a

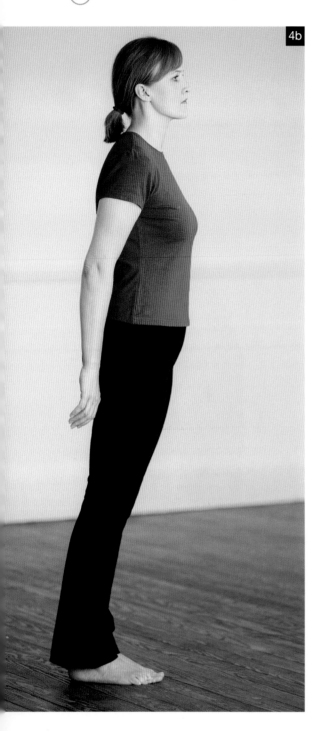

4b

Remember *Pivot at the nodding joint (atlanto-occipital joint), ease the head slowly upward then move it back down more quickly.*
Avoid *Do not lift the head forcefully, arch the back, fix the hips, push air out vigorously or gasp.*

5. Walking breaststroke

The combination of the stepping practice from lesson 1 and the previous nodding practice enables you to integrate the breathing pattern with the stroke before having to negotiate the more tricky transition between water and air.

- Breathe in lightly, begin to exhale and step forward with the right leg, arms extended, head angled to look towards the floor (count 1, 2, 3) (5a).
- With your weight evenly spread on both feet, raise the head, looking just above the hands and continue to exhale (count 4) (5b).
- Maintain this head position and gently open the arms (5, 6). Watch the hands open and continue with the gentle exhalation, weight still evenly spread (5c).
- Scoop the hands inward (5d) and rise gradually on to tiptoes, shifting your weight to the front foot. With the scooping action, allow air to come in through the mouth (7, 8).
- Bow the head, with the gaze directed towards the floor, and begin to exhale (9). Extend the arms and step forward with the left leg; continue to breathe out (10).

Remember *The head movement leads the arm action; inhale passively through the mouth.*

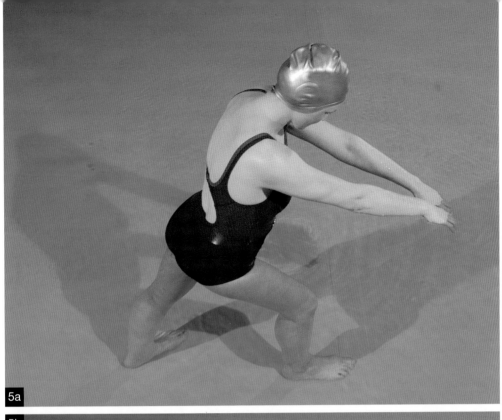

5a

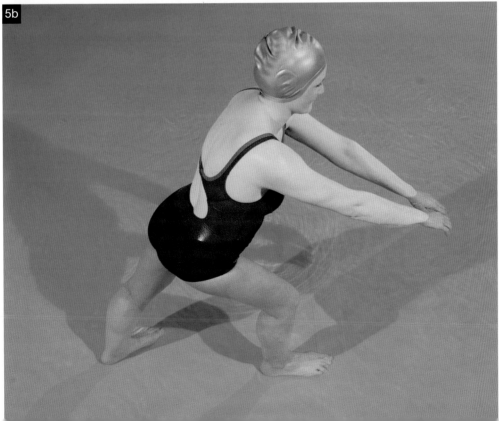

5b

5c

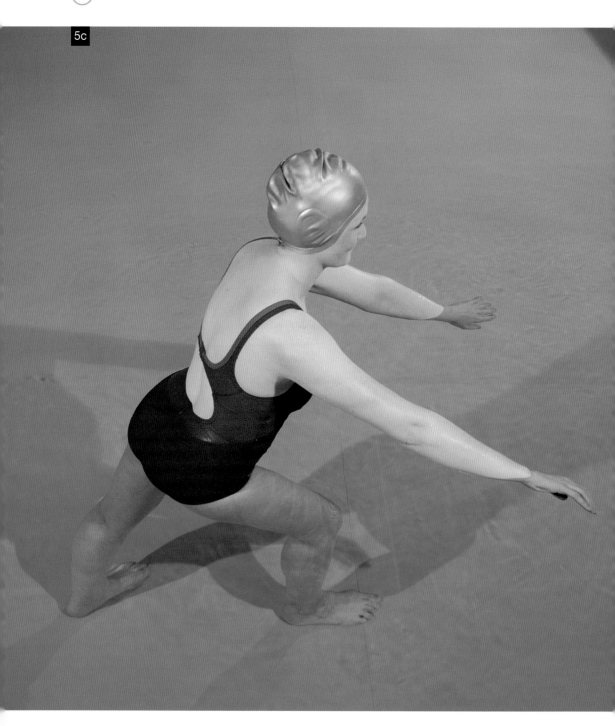

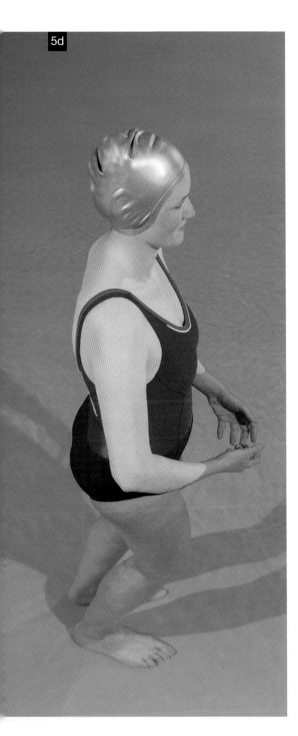

5d

Avoid Do not pull the head back, gasp, look down forcefully or step as the arms open.

6. One complete stroke

This practice coordinates all the elements in one complete stroke cycle. It is helpful to pause at the end of each cycle to focus on integrating the elements.

- Inhale lightly and drift off into a glide with the eyes looking towards the floor (count 1, 2, 3); exhale into the water (6a).
- Continue to exhale as the head rolls, raising the eyes to look just above the hands (4). The nose and mouth remain submerged.
- Widen the back and open the hands (5, 6), still breathing out gently.
- Gently draw the feet drawn towards the seat, raise the head to bring the nose and mouth clear of the water (8); open the mouth and allow the air in (6b).
- Bow the head into the water (9) and start to exhale (6c).
- Extend the legs as the arms reach forward and down into the water (10). Close the legs, maintain a glide for four beats and regain your feet.

Remember Roll the neck before opening the arms. A minimal movement of the head is enough to inhale comfortably. Submerge the face before thrusting the legs.
Avoid Do not lift the head and shoulders too high (the chin should be at the surface on inhalation). Do not breathe in forcefully or break into a second stroke.

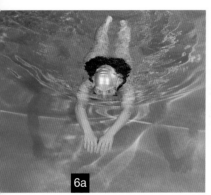
6a

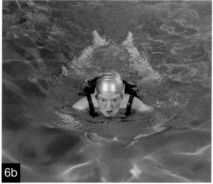
6b

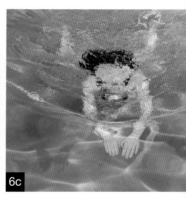
6c

7. Two complete strokes

By producing the action a second time, you gain more awareness of the breathing process. You also experience the wave-like motion that smoothly connects one stroke with the next.

- Inhale lightly and breathe out gently into a glide. Roll the head to raise the eyes, open the hands, scoop with the arms as the pelvis drops with the frog action of the feet, and inhale gently.
- In a continuous movement, bow the head, thrust and close the legs as the arms extend (propels the body forward and down).
- Feel the natural wave-like undulation, allowing the water to lift you before rolling the head and commencing the second stroke.
- Perform one more full stroke, ending up in a long glide, and regain the feet.

Remember Inhale towards the end of the scoop. One stroke flows into the next with head and hips working in concert.
Avoid Do not disturb the head-neck-back relationship, exhale forcefully, tense the pelvis and lower back, or lift the head too high out of the water to inhale.

8. Continuous full stroke

Here are some helpful points to remember when swimming continuously. Think of the breaststroke as a series of glides punctuated by a stroke; the objective is to flow from one glide to the next. When you perform the full stroke it is not advisable to focus on individual elements of it. These are better perfected in the separate practices – here your attention should be on the movement as a whole.

Body orientation: In the horizontal plane, achieve a stable, balanced glide with the neck free and the arms directed down. In the breathing position, ensure that the lower back is released with the eyes looking straight ahead, not upward.
Timing: The propulsive action of the arms in the first part of the action leads you to elevate and inhale, and the thrust of the legs in the second part of the stroke leads you to breathe out as the body is propelled forward and down.

Breathing: Pay attention to the quality of the out-breath, making sure it is gentle and continuous; allow the in-breath to happen by itself. The inhalation only takes a split second, whereas with your face in the water the out-breath is much longer.

Remember Move from one stroke to the next in a consistent and coordinated manner, enjoying the sense of non-doing in the glide. **Avoid** *Do not push air out forcefully. Instead of trying to empty your lungs, deliberately retain some oxygen to make it easier to float to the surface for the next inhalation.*

One complete stroke

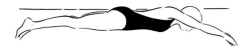

1. Angle the arms downwards, lengthen and widen the back, breathe out gently and look at the floor.

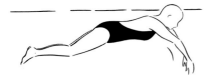

2. Tilt the head with the eyes leading, release the hips, open the arms just beyond shoulder width with elbows slightly bent.

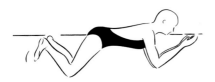

3. Scoop the arms, release the legs and gently draw the feet towards the posterior and passively inhale.

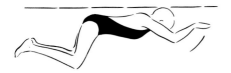

4. Bow the head, thrust with the legs, extend the arms, and exhale.

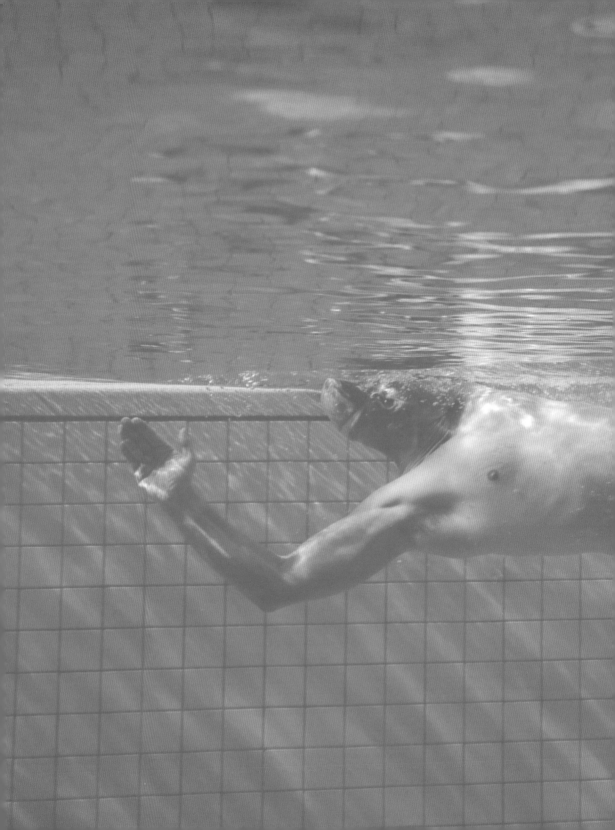

BETTER YOUR BACKSTROKE

'Releasing my hips and shoulders and allowing my head to be supported by the water transformed my back crawl.'

Huseyin Dermis, registered Shaw Method teacher

Throughout the book, the words 'backstroke' and 'back crawl' are used interchangeably to refer to the same stroke.

People have swum on their back since the earliest times: both the Romans and Greeks enjoyed a form of backstroke. The origins of today's backstroke include the elementary backstroke, which involved an overarm recovery and a breaststroke leg action. This inverted form of breastroke was very popular in Europe in the eighteenth and nineteenth centuries, and is sometimes referred to as Old English backstroke.

It was not until the twentieth century that modern-day back crawl was invented. In the 1912 Olympics, Harry Hebner shocked the world when he unveiled this revolutionary way of swimming on the back and beat his rivals by more than three seconds.

The modern back crawl, which has an alternating overarm action and up and down leg action, resembles an upside-down front crawl. Unlike its predecessor, it is an upper-body-dominant stroke, with most of the propulsion being generated by the strong wing-like muscles of the upper back under each arm.

At no point during an effective backstroke is it necessary to submerse the face, and for this reason it helps to build confidence in the water for the less experienced. The head and spine remain centred, with the head fully supported by the water, while the hips and shoulders rotate rhythmically, encouraging free-flowing mobility of the hip and shoulder joints. Success in backstroke can best be achieved by blending the three Rs: relaxation, rhythm and rotation.

Shaw Method key features

Orientation The body rotates to the side, with the hips and shoulders rolling around a central axis – the spine. There is a strong sense of leading with the head, with the emphasis on maintaining stillness through releasing the neck, rather than holding the head still.

Arm action One arm remains extended as the second elevates (not like a windmill). The emphasis is on the thumb leading the arm recovery and the little finger entering the water first. The extended arm leads and assists balance and stability.

Leg action The pace of the leg action is steady, with emphasis on the forward and upward action. The legs are extended while keeping the ankles loose throughout.

Rhythm There are four to six leg beats to every arm cycle. The recovery and anchoring phases are slow, with an acceleration occurring as one arm pushes back and the other enters the water.

Benefits

Swimming on your back benefits postural awareness, promoting a sense of lengthening and widening. As the weight of the head is fully supported by the water, the neck can release easily. Backstroke strengthens the back, tones the legs and arms without putting strain on the spine, and increases hip and shoulder mobility. Many enjoy a feeling of expansion along the sides of the body, which results from the rotational movements. These rotations provide a good base for developing an efficient front crawl. The backcrawl arm action also complements the forward motion of frontcrawl

Risks and common mistakes

Alignment

1. Lifting the head unduly causes strain and increases drag, while letting it fall backwards can give rise to the inhalation of water.
2. If a swimmer does not rotate the hips sufficiently, shoulder mobility is reduced, causing strain and potential injury.

Timing

1. The common pattern of moving both arms at the same time reduces purchase on the water and is a hard habit to break.
2. The breathing pattern is less obvious than in the other strokes, and despite the fact that the face is out of the water, many people have difficulty coordinating their breathing.

Propulsion

1. Failure to release the upper arm before attempting to hold the water can cause a serious injury to the rotator cuff (see glossary).
2. In walking, we are so used to leading with the knees that it is challenging to maintain the length of the leg as it presses upwards.

LESSON 1: ORIENTATION AND LEG ACTION

When swimming on their back, many people enjoy being supported by the water, while others feel a lack of control. Any feelings of uncertainty are compounded by not being able to see ahead. This also makes practice more difficult and increases the risk of injury through collision. This danger is reduced with the Shaw Method as the lead arm is extended for longer periods, leaving the head less exposed.

In the Shaw Method backstroke, the body is on a slight incline, with the head a few inches higher than the hips. This small deviation from the horizontal prevents the legs from breaking the surface. The crown of the head remains in the water throughout; lifting it would cause the hips to sink further, thereby increasing drag. To let the head fall backwards would arch the back and reduce the ability to gain propulsion from the legs. As was discussed earlier, body rotation is vital, reducing resistance and maximizing reach. The following simple practice highlights the relationship between rotation and the movement of the arm in backstroke.

- Stand up for a moment and step straight back with your right foot as you simultaneously extend your right arm behind you. Notice how far the arm extends and be aware of your shoulder joint (photo X).
- Now repeat the practice, only this time rotate your right hip and turn the foot to 90°. See how much further the arm extends without causing any shoulder strain (photo Y).

People float on their back to varying degrees and the main objective of this lesson is to find your optimum point of balance. The head is buoyant, regardless of the way the rest of your body floats, so explore allowing your neck to be free so that the head is fully supported by the water. The other objective is to learn to rotate the torso without disturbing the finely balanced head-neck-back relationship.

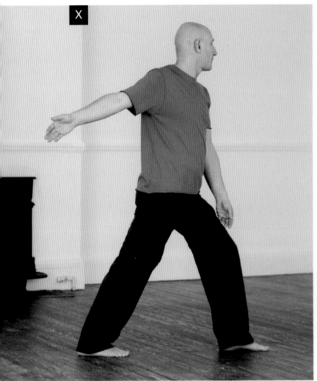

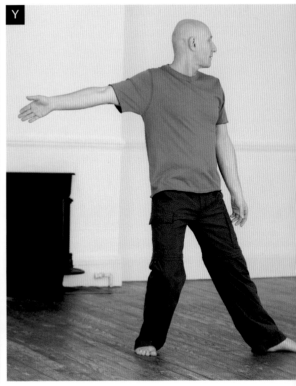

Leg action

The leg action in back crawl is primarily for balance and stability. This movement is generally seen as originating from the hips; however in the Shaw Method, the movement of the legs originates from the lower back. It is important to release the lower back if the hips are to function freely.

Although the arms are dominant in back crawl, the legs still have two important functions: they stabilize the body, providing rhythm, and contribute significantly to forward momentum, generating around 35 per cent of overall propulsion. In the Shaw Method, the alternating action of the legs is described as a 'leg press' (which conveys their true function of maximizing resistance) rather than 'leg kick' (which implies a more forceful, less considered movement).

The leg bends slightly at the beginning of the action and then lengthens as it accelerates upward towards the surface. Turning the feet slightly inward promotes flexibility in the ankles and improves the effectiveness of the leg action, giving greater purchase on the water.

1. Seated leg press

On the poolside you can begin to explore the backstroke leg action and discover when to release and when to apply effort. Observe and feel the effectiveness of moving from the hips as opposed to the knees.

- Sit on the poolside with your eyes looking ahead. Straighten the legs and angle them down into the water. Place your hands behind you as a support and slightly raise yourself, shifting your weight forward.
- Release the left leg so that it is a few inches lower than the right, then bend the knee slightly so the foot drops a little further (1a).
- Straighten the left leg, moving the thigh first, and with toes pointed, actively raise the foot to the surface. The right leg should simultaneously drop a few inches.

- Bend the right knee slightly so that the foot drops a little further. Then actively lift and extend the right leg as for the left.
- Continue the sequence for a minute or two, notice how this action works the stomach muscles as well as the legs.
- Contrast this action with one where you bend the knees to perform a cycling action: notice how much less resistance is generated.

Remember *Make flowing movements, free the ankles, and point the toes. Allow the legs to lengthen.*

Avoid *Do not over-bend the knees, arch or twist the back, or poke the chin forward.*

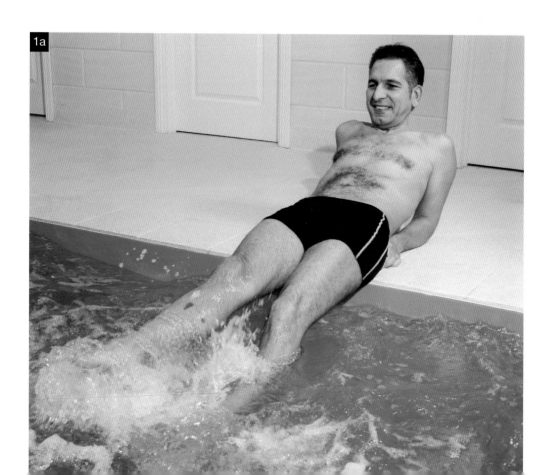

1a

2. Leg action – standing

In an upright stance it is easier to notice how the leg action is affected by your alignment. On the backward release the objective is to reduce resistance and during the forward movement the objective is to maximize it.

- Stand in shallow water by the side of the pool or on a step. Place the left hand on the edge of the pool to steady yourself; the right arm hangs freely.
- Stand tall, on tiptoes, and shift your weight on to the left leg. Eyes at eye level.
- Remaining upright release the whole of the right leg back from the hip joint and slightly bend the knee (2a).
- Extend the right leg forward, pointing the toes and straightening the knee. Notice the resistance of the water as you press the right leg forward until it is slightly in front of the stationary one (2b).
- Repeat this action at least ten times before turning around and performing the action with the left leg.

Remember *Maintain an upright stance and move the leg as a whole, the power being generated through the back and hips.*

Avoid *Do not actively bring the leg back, arch the back, lock the hip or knee, or flex the foot instead of pointing it.*

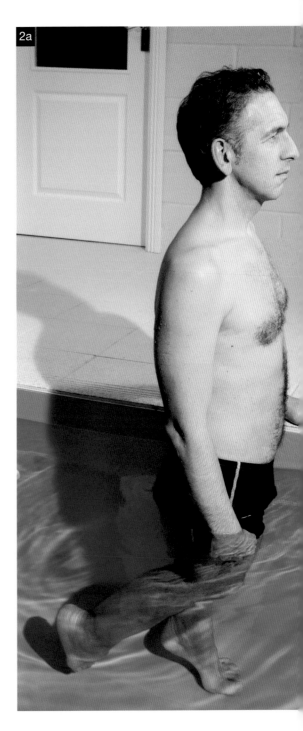
2a

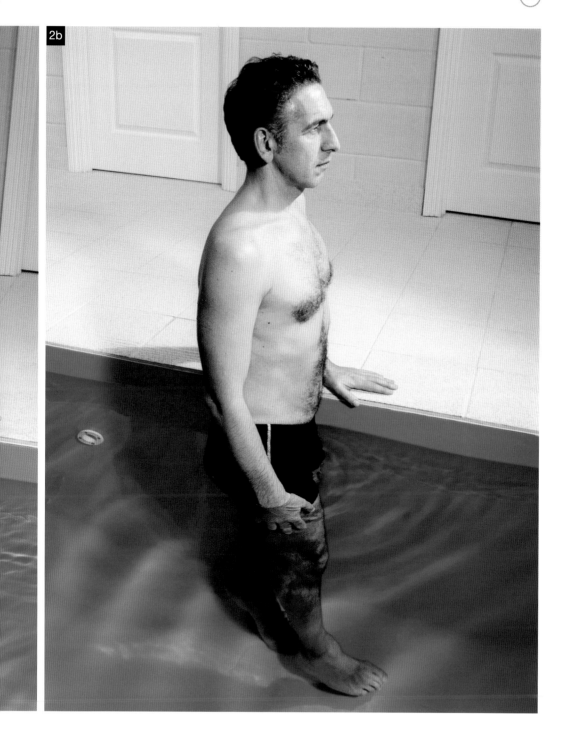

2b

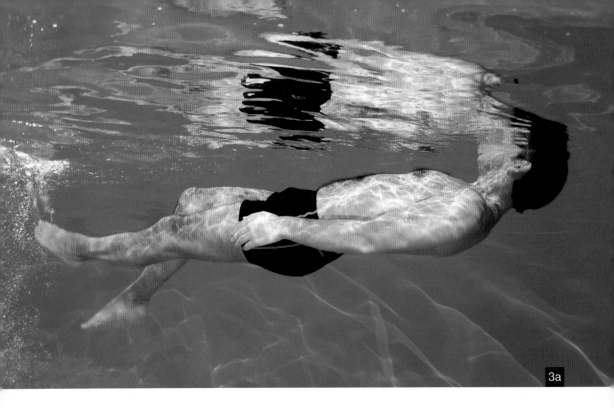

3a

3. Leg action – swimming

This practice builds on the previous one, with the legs propelling the body. In a stable, balanced position, explore how the extended upward beat of the legs generates forward momentum.

- Maintaining good alignment, lower yourself in the water – as if to sit in a low chair – until the shoulders are submerged.
- Slowly lean backwards without poking the chin forward and gradually glide on to the back. Keep your hands by your side, shoulders relaxed, body on a slight incline with head higher than hips, and legs straight with the toes pointed.
- Release the right leg, allowing it to drop a little. Moving the left thigh, press upward with the whole leg. Force is generated through the hips, knees and ankles (3a).
- Notice that as one leg directs upward, the other automatically tends to release downward. Contrast the letting go phase with the more active upward movements.
- Lift the legs alternately and continue for a few minutes. Notice how releasing the neck gives you greater control of this movement. Regain the feet.

Remember *Lengthen the legs as if to lift the water upwards. The downward movement is a gentle release.*

Avoid *Do not rush, lead with the knee or bring the foot out of the water. Do not move your head from side to side.*

4. Sidestepping

The ability to rotate on to the side is fundamental to backstroke. Initially, most people find this orientation challenging, due to a lack of experience in moving side-on. This practice familiarizes you with this new sensation, providing an experience of moving through water in a streamlined way.

- Stand tall with body rotated to the left, head centred and eyes front. Both hands should be resting by your sides with heels together in L-shape (4a).

- With the body still rotated to the side take a small step backwards with your left foot, and simultaneously extend the left arm. Maintain the position of the head. (4b).

- Take a further five or six steps before changing to the other side. Many people feel more at ease on one side; it is a good idea to practise more on the less familiar side.

Remember *Take small steps and maintain balance through good contact with the floor.*
Avoid *Do not move the head up or down or from side to side, hunching the shoulders.*

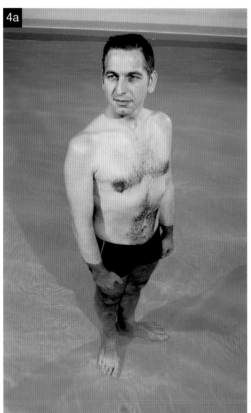

4a

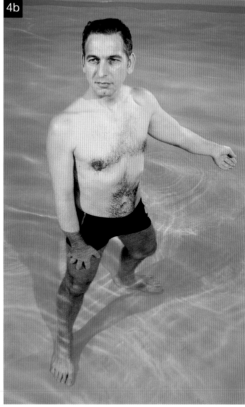

4b

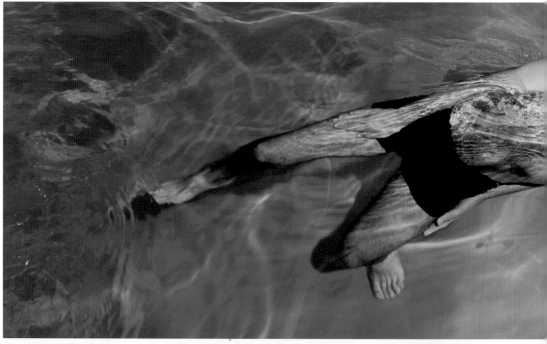

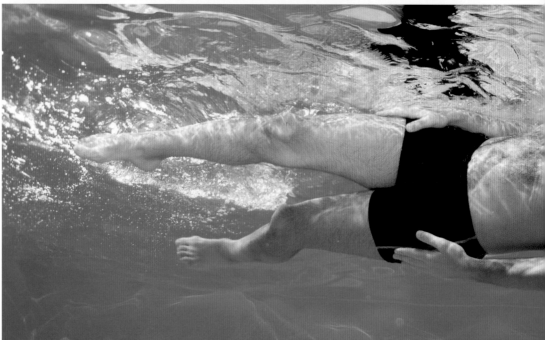

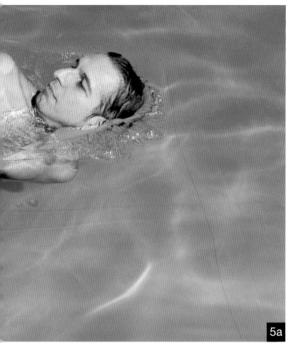

5a

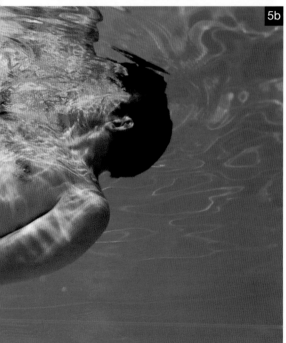

5b

5. Legs to the side

The benefits of streamlining are immediately apparent in this practice, although it is more difficult to balance. The inherent lack of stability in the practice makes it even more important to achieve and maintain a good head-neck-back relationship.

- The eyes face away from the direction of travel. Step backwards with your left foot and rotate your leg and torso outwards (5a).
- Bend the left knee, lowering the head and shoulders towards the surface; arms rest by your sides. Tilt the body so that the right hip and shoulder are uppermost.
- Directing with the head, lean gradually into the water and drift on to your left side with arms alongside the body. Look straight up.
- With your head supported by the water and your body on its side, perform the leg action, actively directing the legs to the right for six beats (5b).
- Roll to a flat position on the back, centre yourself in neutral and regain the feet. Repeat on the other side, noting any differences.

Remember *Keep your neck free, breathing easy, hips and shoulders relaxed, and legs long.*
Avoid *Do not change the head position, kick backwards or lead with the knee.*

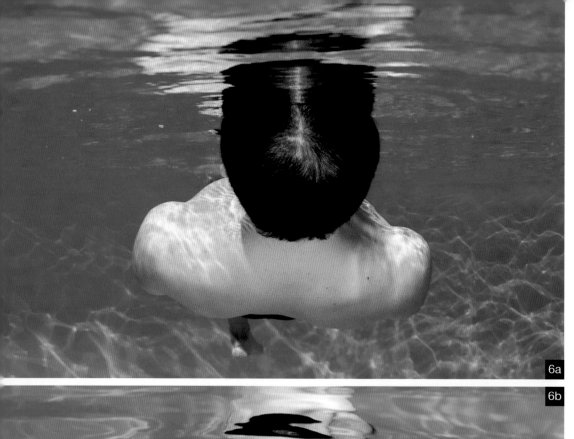

6a

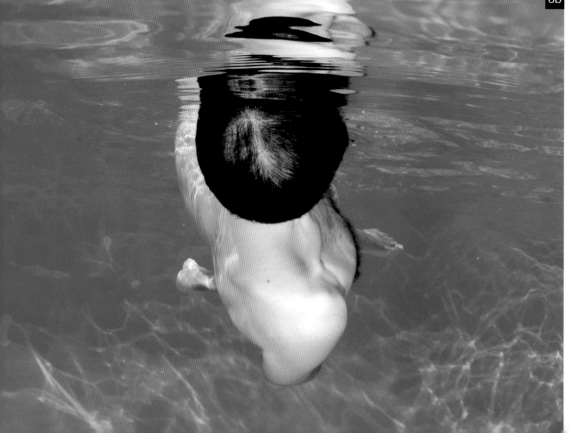

6b

6. Centre to side rotation

Learn to rotate the body without turning the head. Most people automatically turn their heads in tune with the rotation. Freeing the neck is key to a stable head position.

- With shoulders parallel and hands resting by your sides, perform six leg beats (6a).
- Pause the leg action and momentarily direct your gaze upwards. Using the hips and shoulder, rotate on to your right side (6b).
- Continue to move the legs for a further six beats and regain the feet.
- Perform the same series of movements rotating to the left.
- Notice any differences in terms of ability to balance and level of propulsion.

Remember *Make a smooth transition from side to centre, hands and shoulders relaxed.* **Avoid** *Do not allow the head to deviate from the centre-line as the body rotates. Do not lead the leg action with the knee (bicycling).*

7. Arm extended

The objective is to let the arm grow out from the back rather than simply stretch it. Discover how your overall alignment is influenced by the direction of the arm, for example if it veers to the right, the body tends to follow.

- Standing side on, step in the direction of travel with your left leg, and extend your left arm. Bend the knees and gently lower yourself in the water.

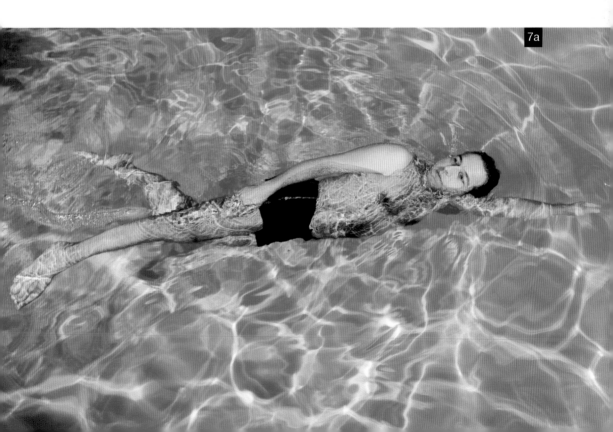

7a

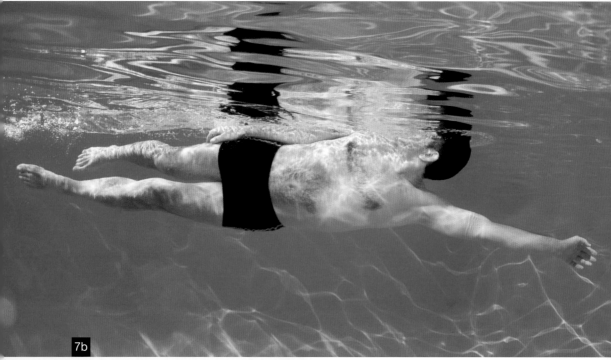

7b

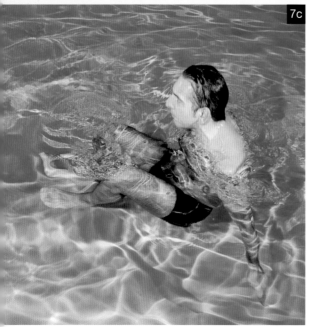

7c

- Leading with the crown, lean into the water and drift on to your side with your gaze directed up, and the lead arm directed forward and angled slightly down (7a).
- The resting arm remains close to your side as if it is placed deeply in a front pocket (7b).
- Maintaining a sideways orientation, perform ten leg beats.
- Draw the lead arm to your hip, roll your body to the centre and regain your feet (7c).

Remember *Think about the arm being connected to the back as an aid to your sense of balance and stability.*

Avoid *Do not let the second arm drift away from your side, as it causes over-rotation.*

LESSON 2: ARM ACTION

Although back crawl is often considered an arm-dominant stroke, it is not actually the arm muscles that generate most of the propulsion. The arms operate as levers connected to the powerful wing-like muscles of the upper back, which provide most of the momentum for driving the body forward.

The arm action consists of four phases: extension, anchor, propulsive, and recovery. An efficient backstroke arm action requires the swimmer to understand when to apply effort and when to release and conserve energy. Most of the effort needs to be concentrated on the dynamic holding phase, with the extension, hooking and recovery phases being significantly less strenuous.

1. Single-arm stepping

By isolating one arm at a time, you can focus on the details of each phase and connect them with the rotational movements of the torso. It is useful to perform it on dry land as well as in the pool.

- **Extension phase** Take a single step backwards with the left leg, turning the foot out as you rotate the body. Simultaneously extend the left arm and direct it down. Ensure that the hand remains soft and is positioned to the left of the shoulder (1a).
- **Anchor phase** Still standing with the right foot leading, bend the left elbow and direct the upper arm away from the shoulder as you move up on to tiptoes with the right foot (1b). Centre the hips and shoulders.

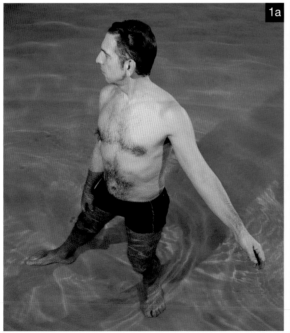
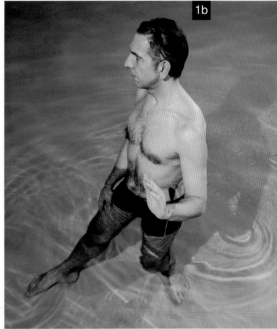

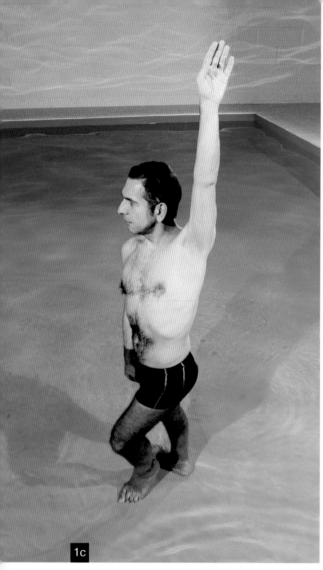

1c

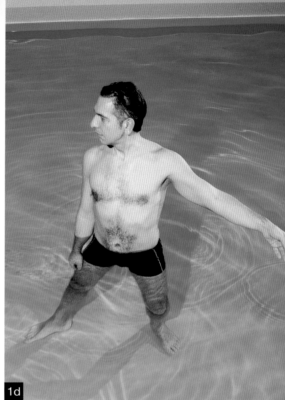

1d

- **Turn and rotate recovery** Turn the hand so that the little finger leads as you continue to make an 180° arc with the left hand, ending up at its start position (extension phase). Simultaneously step backwards with the left leg and rotate the torso to the left (1d).
- Repeat the entire sequence six times and then perform it with the right arm.

- **Propulsive phase** With your left arm parallel to your left shoulder, press it towards the left hip as you step backward and rotate to your right. Ensure that you leave the right arm alone.
- **Recovery phase** Elevate the left arm, leading with the thumb, until it is parallel with your left shoulder; bend the left knee and centre hips and shoulders (1c).

Remember The arm should float lightly through the air. Make smooth, continuous movements of the arms, hips and shoulders. *Avoid* Do not bend the elbow during the recovery, turn and rotate phases. Do not cross the mid-line, move the head or tense the lead arm.

2. Single-arm backstroke

Like the previous practice, the single-arm backstroke brings the focus on to the separate phases of the arm action, in reference to the movement of the rest of the body.

You may be surprised to learn that it is possible to steer a straight course with one arm, as long as the angle of the arm during the propulsive phase is correct.

- **Extension** Launch off with the body rotated and right arm extended in the direction of travel. Look upward as you start the leg action. The left arm rests by your side throughout (2a).
- **Anchor** Bend the right elbow to 90° and flex the wrist as you direct the upper arm away from the shoulder. Simultaneously turn from your side to the centre by rotating the hips and shoulders (2b).

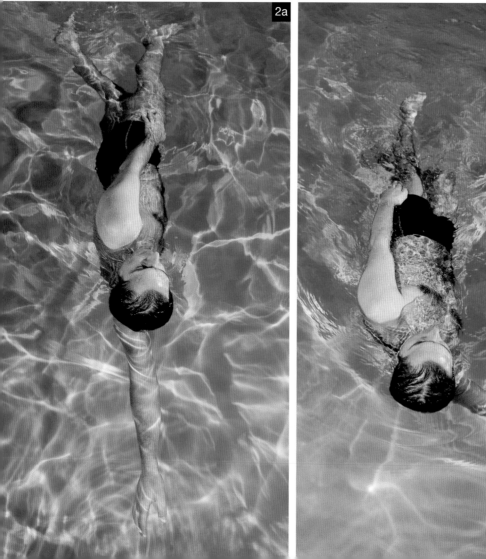
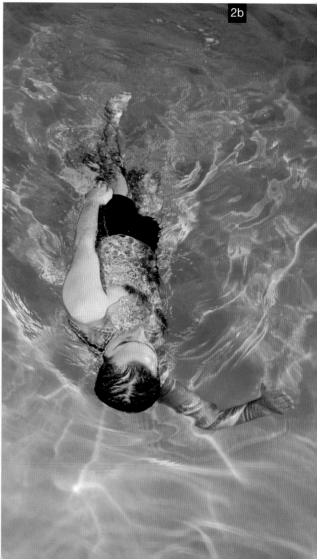

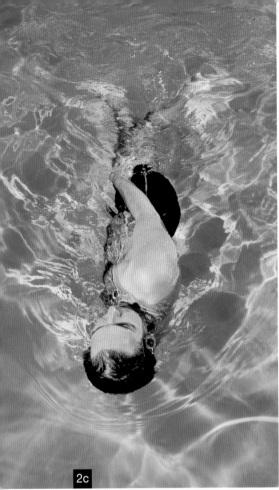

2c

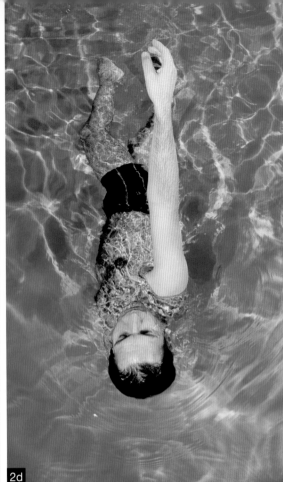

2d

- **Dynamic** Press the right arm in an outward arc and then inward towards the right hip, as the body rotates on to the left side. Accelerate the legs at this point (2c).
- **Recovery** Without pausing, continue to flow into the recovery, exiting the water with the thumb and entering with the little finger as you rotate back to the right side (2d). Repeat the whole sequence with the left arm.

Remember Keep the head still by freeing the neck. Apply force in the pull–push phase. Make the rotations smooth and flowing.

Avoid Do not contract the arm in the hooking phase, bend the arm or cross the mid-line during the recovery.

3. Floating arm – standing (land or water)

This practice establishes the relationship and timing between the arms. It counters the common pattern in which both arms are moved simultaneously like a windmill.

- Starting in neutral, step back, extend the left leg and arm, and lean slightly in the direction of travel.

- **Recovery** Leading with the thumb, slowly raise your right arm until it is level with the shoulder whilst maintaining the length and direction of the left arm.
- In order to remain balanced as the right arm lifts, extend the left arm away in a downward direction.
- Repeat the practice on the other side, noting any differences.

Remember *Imagine that the right arm is growing out from the back as it floats up. Maintain primary control.*
Avoid *Do not lift the shoulders, or shorten the leading arm as the other arm is raised.*

4: Floating arm – swimming

This practice, which corresponds to the first part of the recovery in full-stroke backstroke, cultivates balance and control. It strongly encourages you to make the lifting phase light and to lengthen the lead arm. Lifting the arm with too much effort, or a lack of direction with the lead arm, will tend to push your body down.

- Gently lower yourself into the water with the body rotated to the left and the left arm extended.
- Allowing the head to be supported by the water, launch off on your side with the left arm extended and directed slightly down. Keep the right arm relaxed and close to the right thigh. Start a steady, continuous leg action with the feet close together (4a).
- After ten leg beats leading with the thumb, begin to elevate the right hand slowly and

gently as you consciously extend the left arm, until the right hand approaches vertical above the shoulder (4b). (Those who float lower in the water may find it necessary to perform a vigorous leg action at the point when the arm exits the water.)
- After a further ten leg beats, release the right arm and place the right hand back alongside the thigh. Repeat the whole sequence once again, using the left arm.

Remember *The raised arm is connected with the upper back. Keep the leg action long and loose.*
Avoid *Do not pull the head back and shorten the lead arm as the second is raised.*

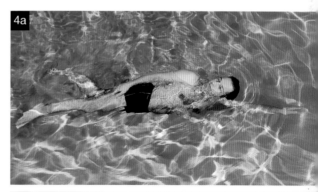
4a

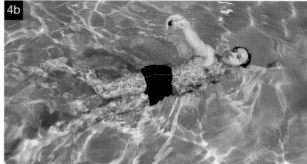
4b

LESSON 3: INTEGRATION

As was mentioned in the overview, one of the most significant differences between the way that most people swim the backstroke and the Shaw Method, relates to the timing of the arm action. The relationship between one arm and the other includes a pause of the extended arm until the second arm has exited the water. This timing enables the swimmer to achieve a good purchase on the water and to maximize the benefit of each propulsive action by swiftly moving into the most streamlined position.

Because the face is continuously out of the water, breathing is often overlooked. In the full stroke, it is important to coordinate breathing with the movement of the arms. I suggest that you inhale on the first part of the recovery, as the thumb leads the arm up to 90°, and exhale as it descends. This is a healthy, comfortable breathing pattern, but if at first it is too challenging, forget about it for the time being and return to it at a later stage.

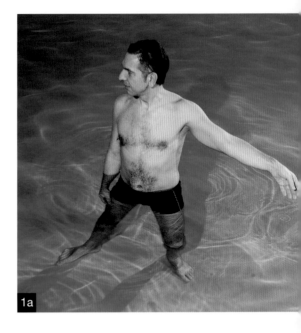

1a

1. Full arm sequence – stepping

Despite the fact that you are standing up rather than on your back, this practice can give you a very similar feeling to swimming full-stroke backstroke. This practice should be performed on dry land first and then in water.

- Stand looking straight ahead, feet apart, body rotated to the left, with your left arm extended (1a). Elevate the right arm, with the thumb leading, until it is level with the shoulder (1b).
- Release the left elbow and direct it away from the shoulder as you turn the torso to the centre. Shift your weight to the left leg and move up on to tiptoe with the right (1c).
- Turn the right palm out so that the little finger leads the up-and-over action as the left arm presses against the water (1d), and the body rotates to the right as the right leg steps back (1e).
- Pause for the count of six and then repeat this complete sequence of actions.

Remember *Concentrate on flowing, continuous transitions, stepping only as the arm comes up and over, i.e. maintain primary control.*
Avoid *Do not move the arms simultaneously (windmilling), or take overly large steps and lose your balance.*

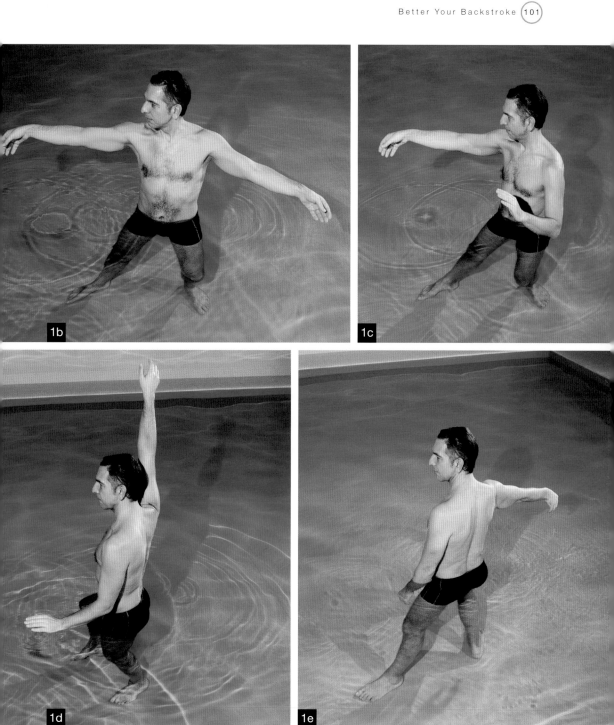

1b

1c

1d

1e

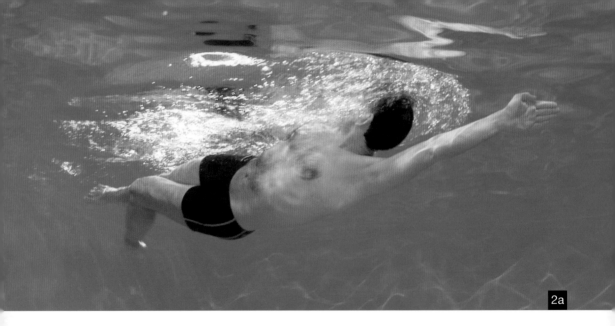

2a

2. One complete cycle

Perform only one complete sequence, to focus on coordinating the arms, legs and torso.

- Step back and out with the left foot, extend the left arm (2a) and lower yourself into a glide with the lead arm extended and the right arm resting on your hip.
- Maintaining the length and direction of the left arm, raise the right arm, leading with the thumb, until vertical.
- Release the elbow and wrist of the left arm (2b), whilst maintaining the position and direction of the right.
- Press against the water with the left arm as the right arm extends (2c) and the body rotates on to the side. The head remains still.

Remember *Flow from one movement to the next without pausing; exit with the thumb and enter with the little finger. Free the neck, allowing the head to be fully supported by the water.*

Avoid *Do not hold your breath, try to push before you bend the elbow, or windmill with the arms.*

3. One cycle followed by six leg beats

This practice gives you the opportunity to focus on your balance and direction and reinforces the lessons on the leg action covered earlier.

The downside of this practice is that the lack of momentum in the recovery, due to the pause in the arm cycle, can make the recovery feel a bit heavy.

- Drift on to your back, with your arms by your sides. Without altering the position of the head, rotate the body to the right and extend the right arm forward under the water.
- Raise the left arm to 90°, maintaining the length and direction of the right arm.
- Release the right wrist and elbow and move into the anchor phase.
- Turn the left arm, and hold on to the water

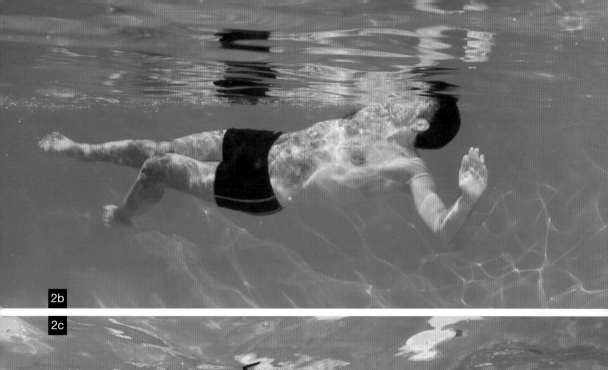

2b

2c

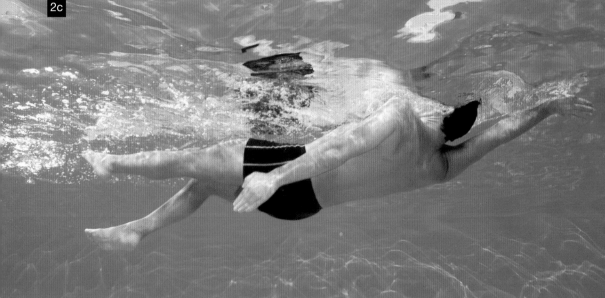

with the right arm as you roll on to your left side and extend the left arm.

- Maintain this position for six leg beats before raising the right arm and repeating the sequence with the left arm leading.

Remember *Hold the water with the right arm and extend with the left. Focus on the quality of the leg action and the head-neck-back relationship when the arms are pausing during the legs-only phase.*

Avoid Do not move the arms simultaneously, hurry the arm or leg action, allow the arms to enter too close to the head, or cross the mid-line underwater.

4. Walk four, swim four

This practice combines the stepping practice you did at the beginning of this lesson with four continuous strokes. By combining walking with swimming, it establishes the rhythm and pace of the stroke. Avoid the mistake of many of my pupils, which is to noticeably increase their pace when they move from the stepping part to the swimming part.

- Perform four complete steps, with the complete arm action, as in the first practice of this section.
- After the fourth step, lower the body and drift off, ensuring that the lead arm is fully extended and the head is centred.
- Perform four complete strokes, as in the previous practice, without compromising the head-neck-back relationship. Regain the feet.
- Stand at full height and move into the stepping sequence, repeat both elements of this practice until the tempo of the walking and swimming are the same.

Remember Flow from the stepping into the swimming, with smooth, relaxed movements. *Avoid* Do not move the arms simultaneously, or Increase the tempo or level of effort in the swimming phases.

5. Integrating the legs with the arms

This practice is designed to help you match the rhythm of the legs with the pace of the arms, and to counter the tendency to over-kick or move the legs too rapidly. The rate can vary between two, four and six leg beats per arm cycle.

- Lower yourself into the water and drift off with your head supported by the water and both arms resting by your sides.
- When you feel stable, start the leg action. Keep the legs long and direct them in an upward direction.
- Rotate the body to the side, slide the right arm under the water, pause for a couple of seconds and then start the arm action.

Remember The right arm and left leg extend simultaneously and vice versa. In the extension phase, notice a diagonal line running from the big toe to the thumb of the opposite hand. *Avoid* Do not arch the back, lead with the knee or rush the leg action.

6. Full stroke – continuous action

- After completing all the previous practices you are ready to swim the full stroke. Instead of pausing the arm action at the end of every cycle, continue in a flowing action. In backstroke the face is permanently out of the water, which can give rise to an irregular breathing pattern. A relaxed, well-balanced stroke requires steady, consistent breathing. See the following list of things to think about and avoid.

Remember *The recovering arm leads the action. Hips and shoulders roll around a constant axis: the spine. Maintain a still head by freeing the neck.*

Rotate the torso so that when the left arm enters the water the right hip and shoulder are on top and vice versa.

In the underwater phase of the arm action, remember to bend the arm and hold the water rather than performing a windmill when the arms lose their grip on the water.

Light recoveries help you maintain a good body position and easier breathing pattern. Allow inhalations to be passive and soft.
Avoid *Do not fix the neck and try to hold the head still. Do not move both arms at the same time. Do not move the arms or legs too quickly, or move the arm in the water too early and/or drop it too deep.*

If you are of average height, the hand should never be lower than about 4 inches (10cm) below the surface.

One complete stroke

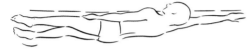

1. Extend one arm with the body rotated, neck free. The leg action balances body.

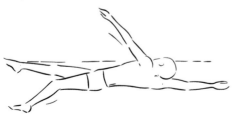

2. Elevate the second arm, maintain the length of the lead arm and rotate the torso to the centre.

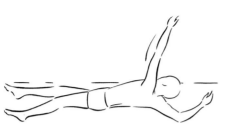

3. Bend the elbow and flex the wrist of the lead arm as second arm moves towards the water leading with the little finger.

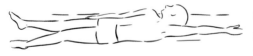

4. Hold onto the water with the lead arm as the recovering arm dynamically extends and the body rotates to the opposite side.

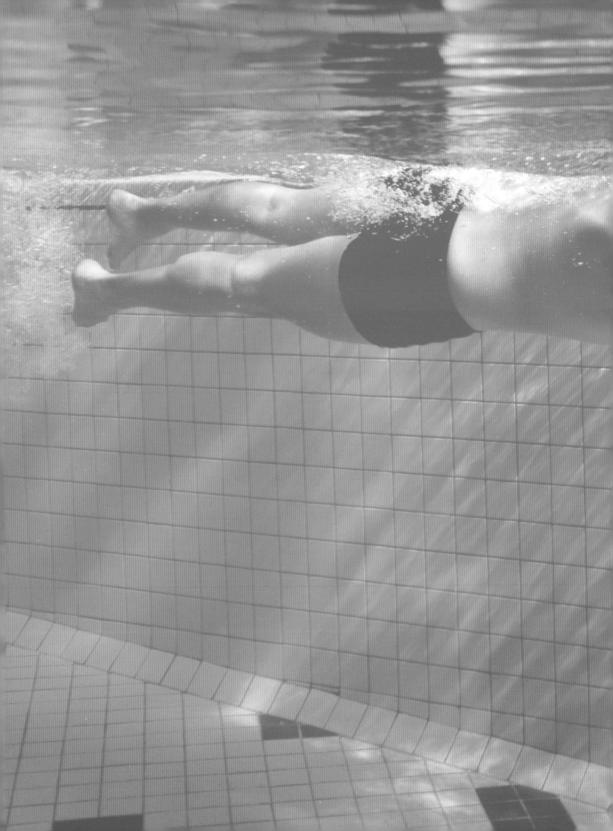

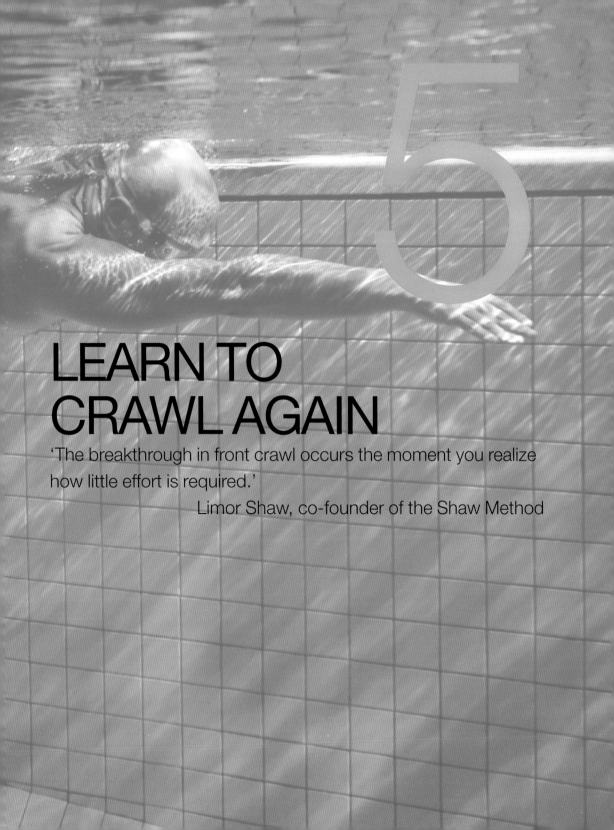

LEARN TO CRAWL AGAIN

'The breakthrough in front crawl occurs the moment you realize how little effort is required.'

Limor Shaw, co-founder of the Shaw Method

A forward-facing, overarm way of swimming has existed since the earliest times. An ancient Egyptian mural (c.1200 BC) clearly depicts soldiers in pursuit of their enemy using a crawl-like swimming action. There is also evidence that the Greeks and Romans swam in this way.

The term 'front crawl' was first coined in Australia in 1893, when a swimming coach witnessed a young boy named Alick Wickham speeding through the water using a stroke that he had never seen before and exclaimed, "Look at that kid crawl." Alick had learnt the stroke from his older brother who, on a visit to the Solomon Islands, had observed locals performing this stroke.

This crude form of front crawl was developed and popularized by two Australian brothers, Syd and Charles Cavill, who took the stroke to Europe and the United States in 1902. It is an interesting coincidence that F. M. Alexander took his technique from Australia to England around the same time. The superior speed of 'Australian Crawl', as it was dubbed, caused something of a sensation. Although it has developed significantly over the last century, the basic principle of combining an alternate, overarm action with a vertical kick in a prone position remains the same. Front crawl is a front-wheel drive stroke, with the arms and upper body providing around 80 per cent of overall propulsion.

In many ways, it is the most intuitive of strokes: a newborn baby will instinctively 'doggy paddle' in a form of underwater front crawl. Swum skilfully, front crawl – with its continuous arm action, streamlined body position and above-water arm recovery – is not only the fastest but also the most energy-efficient of strokes. For this reason, it is generally the stroke of choice for those keen to swim quickly or cover a significant distance. English Channel swimmers, as well as triathletes, invariably choose front crawl. In freestyle competitions, any stroke is allowed but due to its relative advantages over other strokes, almost everyone chooses front crawl.

The easiest of strokes?

Front crawl, the most ergonomic of the four traditional strokes, has many advantages and despite common misconceptions, it is not difficult to learn. The frontal position allows the arms a full range of movement. Coordinating the arms and legs is relatively straightforward. The overarm recovery reduces drag, in contrast to the underwater recovery of breaststroke.

As with the other strokes, front crawl can do more harm than good without body awareness and good technique. **It is not the stroke you swim, but the way that you swim it that counts**.

Shaw Method key features

Alignment The body roll in front crawl is vital, with hips and shoulders rotating around a central axis. The eyes look slightly ahead when the face is immersed, and in the transition between water and air, the head is directed forward while turning to breathe.

Arm action Efficient crawlers spear the arm down into the water, with the elbow and forearm following the hand, which minimizes drag and maximizes stroke length. A bent elbow directs forward prior to the propulsive movement, with the emphasis on holding the water, not on pulling back. The arm recovery is long and light, allowing the elbow to bend as a result of gravity.

Leg action The pace of the leg action is steady and even, with the emphasis on letting go before driving the leg forward, keeping the ankles mobile throughout.

Timing The extended arm remains straight until your recovering arm begins to enter the water. There are two leg beats to every arm cycle unless you are sprinting.

Benefits

Front crawl has many health benefits. It strengthens the back, tones the arms and legs, increases the mobility of the shoulders and hips as well as improving cardiovascular fitness. There is evidence that the alternating action of the left and right side of the body balances the opposite hemispheres of the brain.

Risks and common errors

Alignment

1. Swimming the crawl with the head held high and lifting it to breathe increases drag and strains the neck and back.
2. The traditional high elbow recovery in crawl puts undue tension on the shoulders, which can lead to a form of tendonitis (see glossary).

Timing

1. Most people automatically pull their extended arm back whilst the recovering arm moves through the air (windmilling). This does not produce an effective hold on the water.
2. Many waste a great deal of energy by moving the legs too quickly. A slower, steadier rhythm is more appropriate if you wish to swim for more than a couple of lengths.

Propulsion

1. Many people pull their arms straight back in the water, rather than bending the elbow and flexing the wrist to achieve a more effective anchor before applying propulsive force.
2. The common practice of actively kicking the legs out of the water, employed by many swimmers, can strain and injure the lower back.

LESSON 1: ORIENTATION AND LEGS

A birds-eye view of the Shaw Method front crawl, disregarding the movement of the limbs, reveals that the torso rotates rhythmically from the centre to the side and back again. These changes in body position enable a swimmer to combine the benefits of an effective purchase on the water with streamlining in a way that promotes freedom of movement in the joints.

The objective of this lesson is to feel at ease in the various positions and then to manoeuvre comfortably between them. Here you will learn to employ the leg action and hip roll to balance and achieve these transitions smoothly. Throughout the horizontal practices in this lesson, including those where the body rotates, the head remains still with the face immersed.

Leg action

The leg action of the front crawl aids buoyancy and balances the arm action. Many front crawlers waste energy frantically kicking their legs up and down. In the Shaw Method, the legs' main function is to provide stability and rhythm, although they do produce some forward momentum (around 20 per cent) which assists the all-important body rotations.

The legs alternate: one actively presses downwards while the other releases upwards. This action originates in the lower back and moves through the hip, followed by a small bend of the knee, which then straightens as the whole leg travels downwards. The ankles remain free with the toes pointed throughout; turning the legs slightly inward (in-toeing) produces more even resistance.

Throughout the world, floats are commonly used for practising the leg action. They are not, however, used in the Shaw Method as they compromise alignment and can put pressure on the neck and back. They also create an artificial body position, which is very different from that of the full stroke. It is preferable to direct the arms into the water and work with your own level of buoyancy. Perform the leg action practices in shallow water initially, so that you can stand up comfortably each time you require a breath.

1. Glide

For all the strokes that involve putting the face in the water, we always start with gliding (1a) and the leg press. Acclimatize to the element of water, slow down, and work on your breathing and head-neck-back relationship. For a complete description of the forward glide, see Fun-da-mentals (page 42). Gliding is not only beneficial at the beginning of each stroke session, it is also a useful way of reconnecting to a sense of stillness and being able to let go when working through intricate or challenging practices.

2. Leg press

This standing practice gives you a good sense of how the hip, knee and ankle joints all

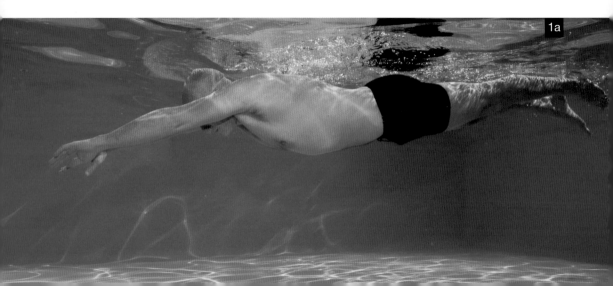

1a

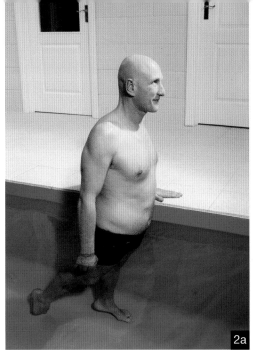

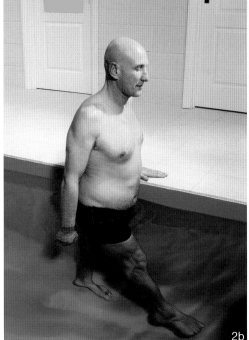

combine in an effective leg action. Moving one leg at time, you can explore the sensation of consciously releasing the leg and actively pressing it forward.

Like the equivalent practice in backstroke, the leg press works on the relationship between alignment and the quality of the leg action. It also highlights a couple of significant differences in the range of motion: in front crawl the knee bends less in the non-propulsive release and the whole leg extends further forward in the propulsive movement.

- Stand tall on your left foot, place one hand on the side to stabilize yourself and move up on to your tiptoes.
- Relax the right ankle, knee and hip, and release the leg backwards, so that the upper thigh and foot are behind the left leg (2a).
- Extend the right foot, straighten the leg

without locking it and swing the whole of the leg forward so that it is positioned in front of the left (2b).

- The movement starts in the hip and finishes with the foot pointing at an angle down and away from the body.
- Repeat this action six times before alternating legs.

Remember *Stand tall throughout. On the back swing, maintain the length of the leg and head-neck-back relationship. You should feel minimal resistance on the backward action and strong resistance on the forward action.*

Avoid *Do not arch the back when you release the leg backwards. Do not move the leg too wide so that you lose your balance, or move the head up or down or from side to side.*

3. Front leg action

By translating your understanding from the previous practice (of when to release and when to apply effort) to the horizontal plane, discover how the legs generate forward momentum.

- Step forward as you extend both arms and smoothly drift into a stable, balanced glide; breathe out gently.
- Release one leg upward and actively press the other (lengthened) leg down into the water (3a).
- Notice how, as you actively press down with one leg, the other rises passively.
- Perform 6–10 leg beats before regaining your feet.

Remember *Release the lower back, hips, ankles and knees. In-toe slightly on the forward action. Aim for a fluent, flowing action.*
Avoid *Do make stiff, 'wooden' kicks, bend the legs too much or bring the feet high out of the water. Do not push harder with one leg than the other, actively blow out air, or hold your breath.*

4. The fencer

This practice gives you an experience of moving through water with minimal resistance. It is a comfortable and secure introduction to moving through the water on your side, and connects the lead arm with the powerful muscles of the back.

- Stand with your right foot facing forward and the left turned out, with the heels together at right angles and your weight evenly spread. Keep your hands by your sides and look straight ahead (4a).
- Step forward with your right leg, extending the right arm with the thumb uppermost, arm angled downward; leave the left arm alone (4b).
- Draw your left leg towards the right, bringing the heels together and the feet at right angles to each other. Release the right arm to rest by your side.
- Centre your weight before stepping forward with the right leg and extending the right arm again. Repeat four times before leading with the left leg, noticing any differences.

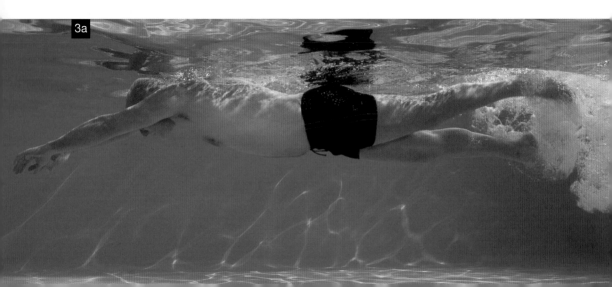

3a

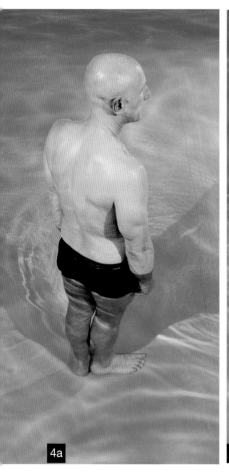

4a

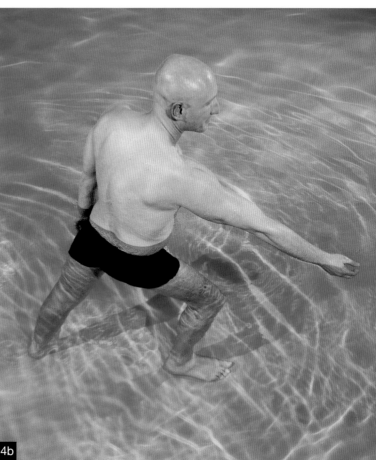

4b

Remember *Maintain a steady rhythm, allowing the arm to grow out from the back, and keeping the neck free and the head centred.*
Avoid *Do not cross the mid-line with arms or legs, step outside hip width, or move the head from side to side.*

5. Side kick

In this practice on the side, although it is more challenging to balance, you immediately experience how frontal resistance is reduced,

easing forward movement. It also provides an opportunity to develop your balance on both sides. At first, most right-handers tend to find it more comfortable to lead with their right arm, and vice versa.

● Step forward with the left leg, extend the left arm and drift on to your side, breathing out gently into the water (5a).
● The body balances on its side with head centred and eyes looking down.

- In this rotated position, start a slow, even leg action directing the effort towards the right side for 6–10 leg beats.
- Roll back to the centre and regain your feet.
- Repeat the practice leading with the left arm, noting any differences.

Remember *When the right arm leads the movement, legs kick to the left and vice versa.*
Avoid *Do not commence the leg action before you are balanced on the side. Do not arch the lower back and/or over-rotate.*

6. Centre to the side

Many people find it relatively straightforward to keep their head still when they are on their side or in a flat position, but most find it much more of a challenge when these two orientations are combined. By focusing on the direction of travel you will find it easier to keep the head centred.

- Glide with both arms extended, palms facing downward, and hips parallel.
- Once you are stable on your front, begin the leg action, performing it for six beats before pausing in preparation for the transition (6a).

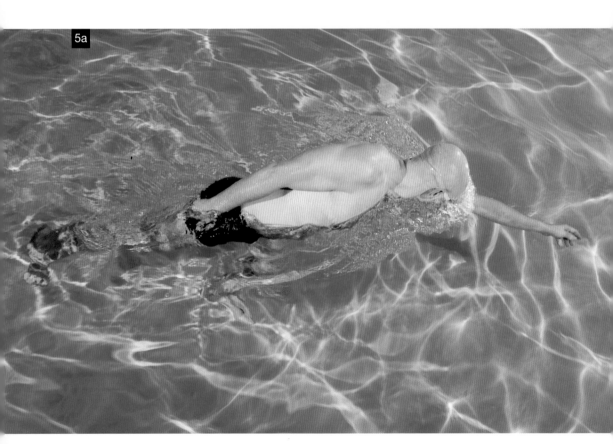

5a

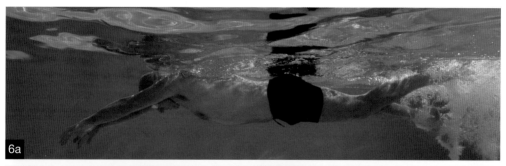

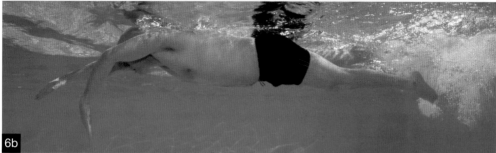

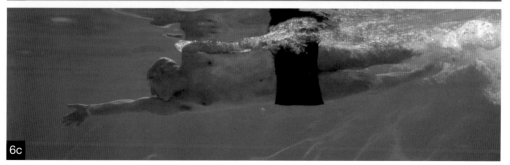

- Release the elbow and wrist of your left arm so that it is crooked (6b). Draw it towards the left hip; simultaneously direct the right arm forward.
- As the right arm extends, spiral it forward and down into the water. Turn the rest of the body from the hips to the left side. The head remains centred with the eyes looking slightly forward (6c).
- Perform the sideways leg action for six leg beats, centre the body and regain the feet. Perform the sequence again, ending up with left arm leading.

Remember *Neck free and shoulders and hips roll around a central axis. Feel as if you are swimming downhill.*
Avoid *Do not turn the head as you rotate, shorten the lead arm, snatch the other arm back, or hold the breath.*

7. Side – centre

This practice, the reverse of the previous one, gives clear and immediate feedback on the way that the angle of the body affects forward movement. The resistance of the water makes the process of recovering the arm a little tricky; applying less effort makes this movement easier. This same principle applies in the full-stroke recovery, where many waste effort.

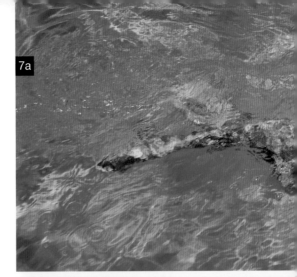

- Drift on to your side, with the left arm leading. Once stable, start the leg action to the side and continue for six beats (7a).
- Pause the legs, release the wrist and elbow of the right arm and sweep forward as if performing an underarm bowling action, until it is parallel with the left arm, and the body is gliding flat with both palms down (7b).
- When both arms are parallel, shoulder-width apart, and the body is stable, restart the leg action for six beats before regaining the feet (7c).
- Repeat the practice, this time starting with the right arm.

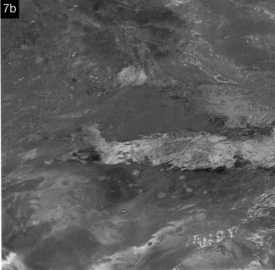

Remember *Free the neck, particularly in the transition. Maintain the direction of the lead arm as you move to the glide.*
Avoid *Do not apply excessive effort as you move the back arm parallel with the front – it will push you back. Do not pull the head back and raise your eye level.*

8. Crawl rotation

Once you are comfortable making the transition from centre to side, and side to centre, you can

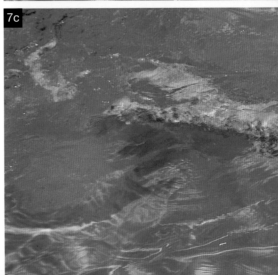

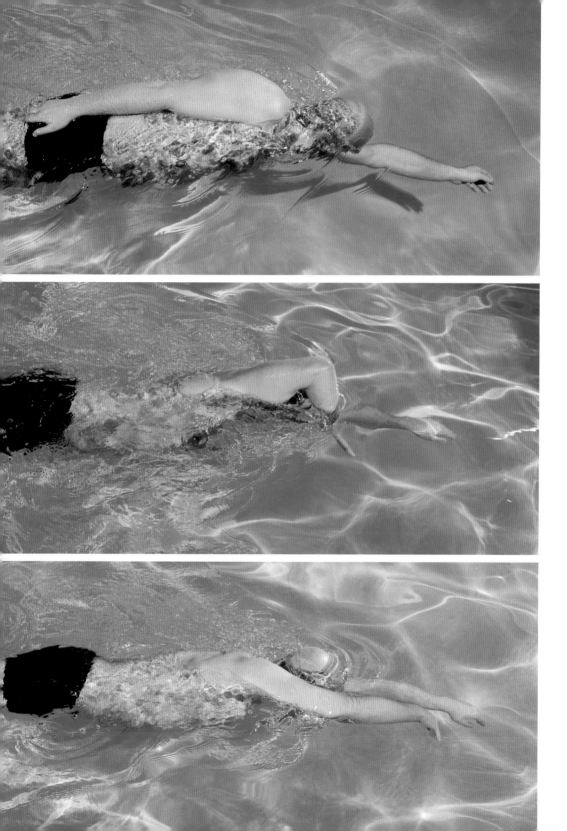

combine the two in a single practice. Here the emphasis is on thinking forward and maintaining a central head position as the body changes orientation. Depending on your lung capacity, rotate after every four or six leg beats. Fitter and more confident swimmers will choose the latter.

LESSON 2: ARM ACTION

The overarm actions in the back and the front crawl share many characteristics, the arms and upper body generating most of the propulsion. In Shaw Method front crawl, the lead arm maintains its length until the recovering arm begins to enter the water. This aids stability and improves purchase. The emphasis is on using the arms to hold the water, as if you were pulling yourself along an imaginary rope rather than trying to pull back. The torso effectively passes the anchored arm.

Do not be surprised if at first you find this new sequence challenging, as it goes against a natural inclination to swing both arms at the same time. Spend time establishing this new movement pattern on dry land before taking it into the water, because when you swim the stimulus to revert to habit is invariably stronger.

The arm action has five phases: extension, anchor, propulsive, salute and handshake. This lesson teaches the phases separately and then you link them together in a flowing way. It is important not to think of the arms working in isolation.

In this lesson, you will explore how head position, the movement of the torso and the leg action all have a major impact on the quality of the arm action. Similarly, the way you hold your hands also has a significant impact. Many people are accustomed to swimming the crawl with tense hands: they often falsely believe that by stiffening them they will get more purchase on the water. Experience shows that supple and open hands are always more effective.

When learning to coordinate arm movements with the rest of the body, it is vital that the head remains centred. Exhale gently whenever the face is submerged; the more you exhale, the lower your body tends to sink and the more effort is required to propel yourself forward. Having a reserve of air in your lungs not only helps you to remain relaxed and focused but also increases your buoyancy.

The distinctive Shaw Method front crawl arm recovery resembles the wings of an eagle, as opposed to the traditional high elbow recovery commonly known as 'chicken wings'. Our eagle-like arm action is streamlined and powerful. Because it does not involve hunching, it minimizes strain on the shoulder joint.

1. Single-arm stepping

This practice can be performed in the pool or on dry land. Being upright, you have a clear view of the arms in four of the five phases, which makes coordination easier. Work on each phase separately before linking them together in a flowing way. You may find it helpful to perform the practice in front of a mirror.

Extension – palm down

● Stand with your left foot pointing forward, right turned out, heels together in an

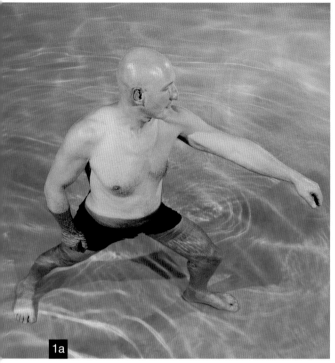

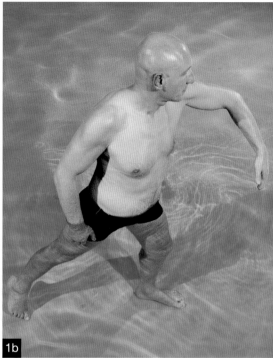

L-shape, body rotated to the right, arms by the sides. The head is centered, looking ahead.

- Step forward with the left leg and simultaneously extend the left arm with the palm down.
- The fingers are below the wrist, wrist below the elbow, elbow below the shoulder. Both feet are firmly on the floor. Leave the right arm resting by your thigh (1a).

Remember *The arm grows out from the back, engaging the muscles of the upper back.*
Avoid *Do not lock or hyper-extend the leading arm, lift the shoulder, tense the back arm, or pull the head back.*

Anchor

- Flex the wrist and elbow and rotate the forearm so that the fingers are pointing down and the elbow is directed forwards.
- Lengthen from the shoulder to the elbow as you shift your weight forward and rock up on to the straightening front leg, allowing the heel of the back foot to lift (1b).

Remember *Direct the elbow forward. Maintain balance by keeping the lead foot grounded.*
Avoid *Do not hunch the shoulder as you bend the elbow or look down at the floor.*

Propulsive

- Draw your left arm towards your left hip and

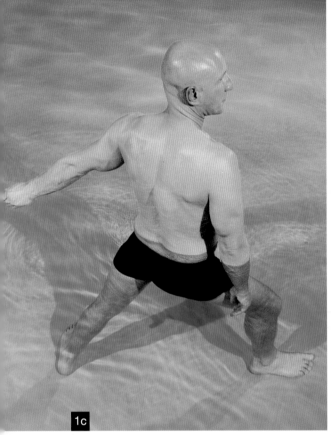

1c

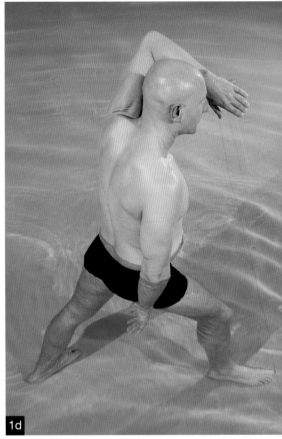

1d

step forward with the right leg.

● Widen the back, rotate the arm and body to
the left as the arm passes the hip, and
extend it behind you with the thumb
uppermost. The head is centred and the
eyes continue to look forward (1c).

Remember *Keep the heel down. Make
smooth transitions from the right arm to the left.*
Avoid *Do not over-rotate the shoulder, narrow
the back, tense the arm or raise the back foot
on tiptoe.*

Salute

● Without pausing, continue the movement of
the left arm up and over and rotate the right
hip back to the centre so that the torso faces
forward, relaxing the chest.

● As the hand reaches the highest point,
release the elbow and allow gravity to bring
the hand down a few inches to the left of the
face, as if to salute, with the palm facing
outwards (1d).

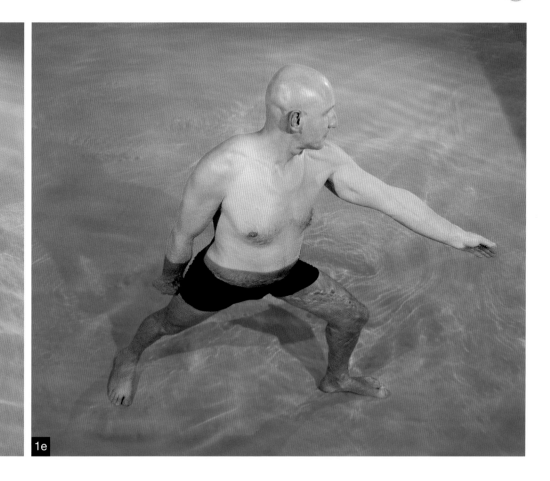

1e

Remember *Your arm grows out from the collarbone. Keep a sense of lightness as the arm flows through the air. Stand tall throughout.*
Avoid *Do not pause in the transition between the third and fourth phases, as this makes the arm heavier. Do not drop or pull the head back.*

Extend to handshake

- As you dynamically step with the left foot and rotate the body without moving the head, spiral the left hand forward and slightly down.

- The hand ends up with thumb on top, as if to shake someone's hand. The arm is fully extended, engaging the upper back muscles in a slight downward trajectory (1e).
- Repeat this complete cycle four times before transferring to the left arm.

Remember *Keep the neck free and head centred throughout. The hand remains relaxed and open.*
Avoid *Do not reach upward or arch the back as the arm extends forward.*

2. Standing start

This practice, with both arms in front, provides a stable base for starting each action. In the early stages it is beneficial to use it in both standing and swimming practices.

- Stand with the heels together in an L-shape, the right foot facing forward and the left turned out. Keep both arms by your sides.
- Step forward with the right leg, simultaneously extend the right arm forward, and raise the left arm up and over into the salute phase (2a).
- Allow both arms to release down to the side and perform the same sequence with the left arm leading, noting any differences.

Remember *Move forward and up. Both arms grow out of a lengthening and widening back.*
Avoid *Do not drop the head, or hunch the shoulder by unduly elevating the elbow.*

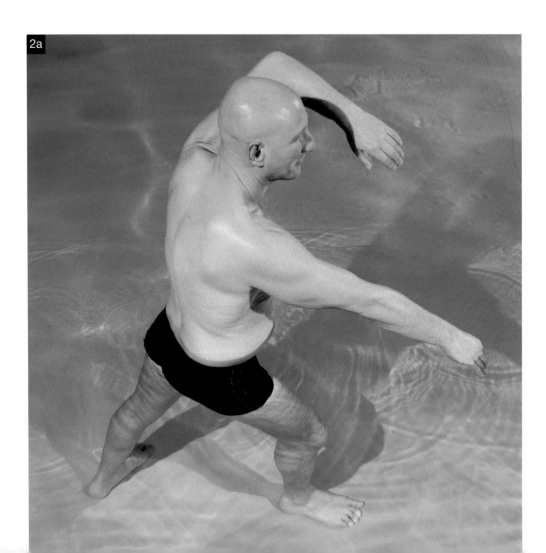

2a

3. Arms stepping

Standing upright, with your face out of the water, allows you to firmly establish this newly coordinated arm action.

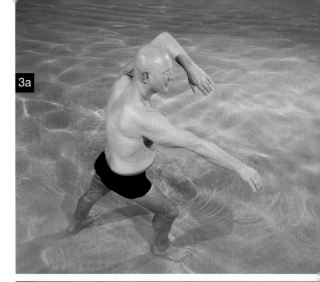

- Step forward with the right leg, lengthen and widen the back, and move the arms into the standing start phase (3a).
- Flex the right wrist and elbow, gently press the hand and forearm down on the water, and shift the weight forward and up into the hook phase (3b).
- Step forward with the left leg, the left arm spiralling into the handshake phase, the right arm releasing back and turning out, with thumbs up. The right foot is turned outward and your weight is evenly spread (3c).
- In a flowing action, let the right arm continue its movement up and over. When it reaches its highest elevation, allow gravity to help it bend into the salute phase; as it descends rotate the left arm so that the palm is face down. Keep your weight centred.
- Release the arms and start the practice again with the opposite arm leading.

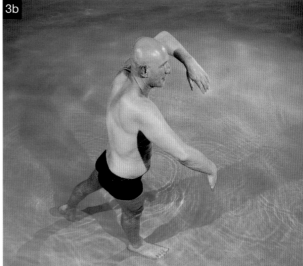

Remember *As the arms move into the extension phase, keep your heels on the floor. Thumbs leading the arm action.*
Avoid *Do not tense the shoulders or contract the upper back. Insufficient hip rotation can strain the lower back. Do not drop the lead arm.*

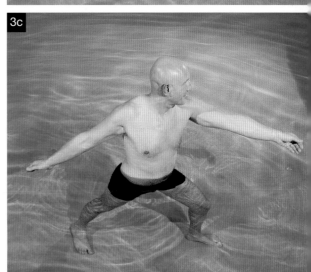

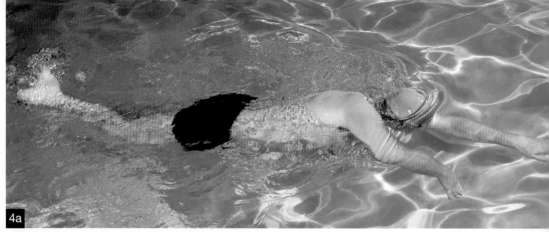

4a

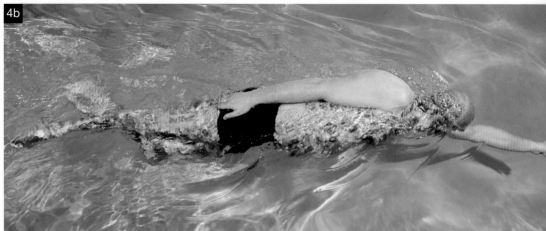

4b

4. One-cycle swimming

Having learned to coordinate the arm action on a vertical plane, you are now ready to apply the action to swimming. The emphasis should be on holding the water and focusing attention on the direction of travel. Many people find it a challenge to complete only a single sequence; do not give in to the temptation to do more.

- Launch into a glide with both arms extended and angled downward.
- Bend the right wrist and elbow to hook the water (4a).
- Achieve purchase on the water with the right arm as the left extends forward into the handshake phase and the body rotates on to its left side (4b).
- Maintain the length of the left arm as the right arm flows straight up (4c) and over into the salute phase, and the body and lead arm rotate back to a flat, centred position (4d).
- Extend into a glide and regain the feet. Then perform a single sequence that starts on the other side.

Remember *The recovery of the arm should be as light as possible, with the neck free throughout.*

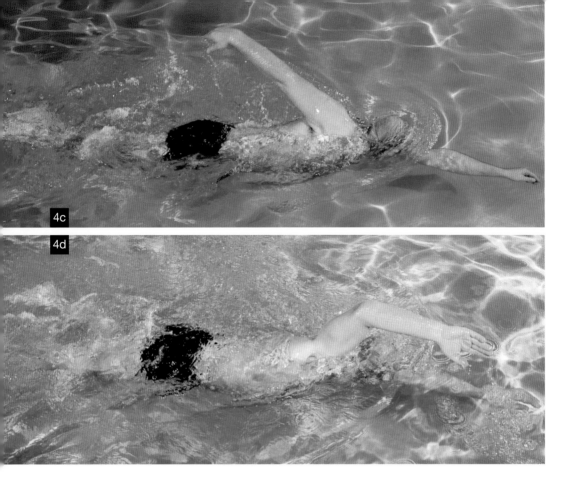

4c

4d

Avoid *Do not raise the head, lose the length of the lead arm or break into a second stroke.*

5. Walk four, swim four

Walking establishes rhythm and pace, which is carried over into the stroke. It is important to count full strokes, i.e. at the point when both arms are forward. If you count when the arm pulls back it confuses the timing and can cause the lead arm to drop.

- Focus on the timing, paying attention to the beginning and end of each cycle – one arm extended; the other in the salute position.

- Establish a slow, steady rhythm for walking, followed by similarly paced swimming strokes.
- Leave the face in the water when swimming, and breathe out gently throughout. Excessive exhalation not only triggers anxiety, it also causes the body to sink lower.

Remember *Breathe out gently. More air is released in the recovery phase, where the recovering arm bears down on the breathing apparatus, than in the propulsive phase (where the arm is below the chest).*

Avoid *Do not speed up the stroke rate when*

swimming. Do not lose the timing, i.e. pull back too early. Do not breathe out forcefully.

LESSON 3: BREATHING WITH EASE

In front crawl, inhalations are made through the mouth by turning the head to the side.

Many people find it hard to understand why, when they were younger, they were able to swim length after length of front crawl, but in later life, after a short distance, they gasp for air. In most cases this has more to do with incorrect positioning and a lack of flexibility than fitness and stamina.

An effective breathing pattern results from having understood and absorbed the essentials of the crawl covered in the previous lessons – if these are not firmly in place, breathing will invariably break down. By building on this foundation, in this lesson you can see how body rotation and a swift turn of the head combine to establish an effective breathing pattern. The rotation provides more room, making the transition between water and air easier. You can also draw on the backstroke skills acquired earlier, as the hip and shoulder roll in back crawl is similar to the breathing position in front crawl. The following dry land practice graphically illustrates the significance of the hip roll in breathing during the front crawl.

- Stand with one foot in front of the other, turn your head to the right as far as is comfortable. Unless you are exceptionally supple, you are likely to feel tension in the shoulder and a lack of space (X).

- Turn your right hip outward so that the right foot is at 90°. Rotate your head to the right, eyes looking slightly up – notice how much further you can turn it and how much more comfortable it feels (Y).

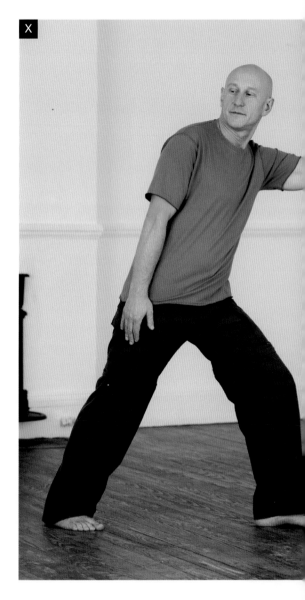

X

We can directly relate this experience to swimming the front crawl. The first position represents turning to breathe without rotating the hip and shoulder, the second to breathing with the body rotation. In the first position, a lack of space makes it almost impossible to breathe without lifting the head and shortening the neck, which inevitably causes the hips to sink and also restricts the lungs. When the body is rotated to the side, the crown stays

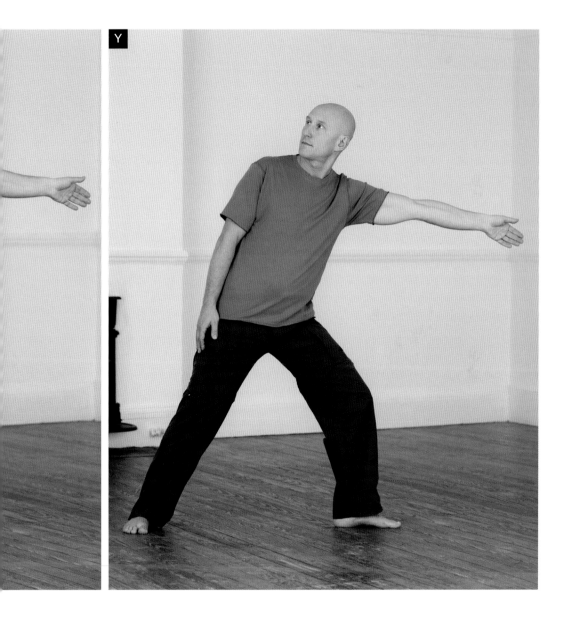

submerged, the neck remains long, and breathing is relatively straightforward.

To achieve an effective transition between the face being in and out of the water, the turn of the head must be integrated with the movement of the arms. In the previous section we explored the importance of maintaining the length and direction of the front arm until the second arm begins to enter the water, in order to promote maximum propulsion. This timing is even more significant for breathing. If the front arm pulls back before the head and recovering arm have entered the water, not only will you fail to gain an effective purchase on the water, but you are also likely to sink and breathe in water.

Bilateral and unilateral breathing

Most people have a favoured side when it comes to breathing: right-handed people usually feel more comfortable turning to the left, and left-handed people find it easier to breathe to the right. However, an efficient front crawl calls for bilateral breathing, taking one breath every third or fifth arm recovery (every 1.5 or 2.5 cycles, depending on lung capacity and fitness level). Opting for unilateral breathing on the more comfortable side is like doing flexibility exercises only on parts that are flexible. Over time, unilateral breathing can have major postural implications, leading to a lack of symmetry. Breathing on both sides also gives a much better sense of flow and rhythm.

The practices in this section work towards bilateral breathing. Initially it is advisable to spend more time on the side you find most challenging. Following the rotational work you did in previous lessons, you may discover that bilateral breathing comes surprisingly easily.

1. Legs to the side

This position is not actually found in front crawl, but is very beneficial for getting comfortable on your side and for discovering how to position the head. It requires a little more rotation towards your back than is necessary in the full stroke.

● Stand with your left foot forward and the right foot turned outward. The head is in neutral, facing forward.
● Take a forward step with the left foot and turn the neck to direct the gaze back and up to the right.
● Slowly descend on your left side until the shoulders are submerged, with the arms resting by your sides. Gently drift off with your face clear of the water (1a).
● Start the leg action: focus on releasing the back and pressing the whole of each leg forward.

Remember Lead with your crown. Both ears are submerged and both eyes out of the water. Release the lower back and allow the legs to move freely from the hips.
Avoid Do not lift the head or one shoulder, sweep the legs too widely or perform a cycling-type leg action.

2. Extending the arm and turning the head

This practice can be performed in the pool or on dry land. It improves the range of motion of the neck and opens out the sides of the body. It

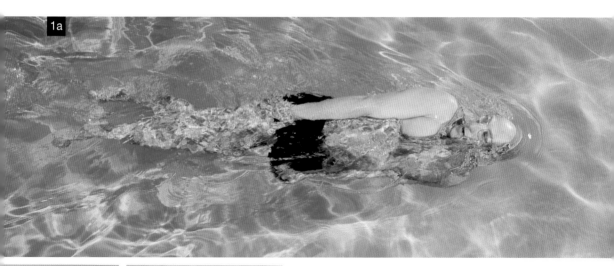

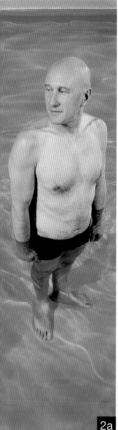

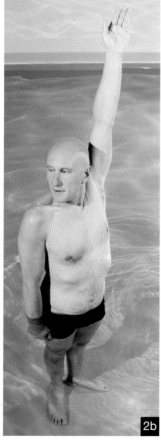

familiarizes you with this new alignment and connects the arms with the back, which is essential for producing a stable foundation from which to breathe.

- Stand tall, with your feet postioned in an L-shape – the right one facing forward and the left one turned outward. Place your arms by your sides and turn your head to look over your right shoulder (2a).
- Extend the left arm directly upwards, as if you were reaching for the sky, and release the right shoulder (2b).

Remember *Release and lengthen the neck and allow the arm to grow out from the back.*
Avoid *Do not arch the back, or fail to extend the arm fully, allowing it to drift off to the side instead of being directed straight up.*

3. Lunge and breathe

This practice takes your upper body on to a horizontal plane and prepares you to launch off into a comfortable breathing position. It is useful to think of your lead arm being firm and stable, and the upper arm being soft and loose.

- Step forward with the left foot, as the left arm extends without lifting the hand higher than the elbow; leave the right arm alone (3a). Shift your gaze by turning the head a little more to the right, to look slightly back and up.

- Perform six leg beats to maintain this position, then bring the right leg forward to the left heel and stand up to full height. Release the right arm so that it rests by your side.

- Perform the sequence again, this time leading with the left leg.

Remember Turn the head smoothly as you lunge forward. Keep the back open throughout. **Avoid** Do not tense the shoulder of the lead arm or lift it towards the ear. Do not look forward just before you lunge. Do not take a large step forward.

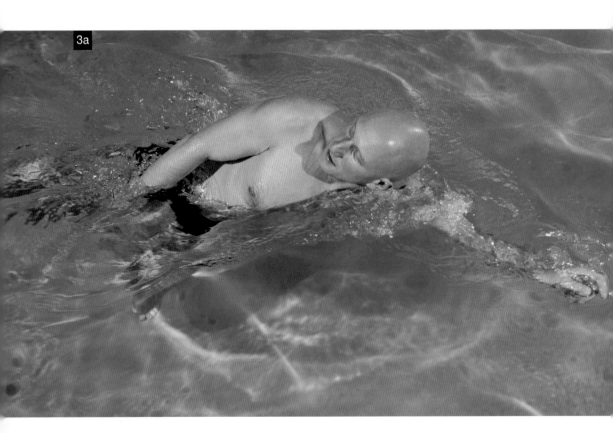

3a

4. Side step to breathe

This practice develops the ability to allow the arm to grow out from the back and acclimatizes you to the feeling of moving through water on your side without being able to see where you are going.

- Start with your feet in an L-shape, hands by the sides, eyes front (4a).
- Lunge with your left foot, extend the left arm at a downward angle. As you step forward, turn the head so that the gaze is directed back and up, and gently breathe in through the mouth (4b).
- Maintain this position for a count of four. Step forward with the right foot, releasing the right arm as you breathe out for a count of six.
- Repeat this sequence six times and then perform it leading with the right arm, noting any differences. Most left-handed people find it easier to turn to the right, and vice versa.

Remember *Breathe in as the arms open, and out as they close. Direct the lead arm away.*
Avoid *Do not hold your breath or breathe in as the arms close. Do not cross the mid-line, twist, or tense the neck.*

5. Leg action – swimming on the side

This practice closely corresponds to the breathing position in full-stroke front crawl. Apart from being an ideal way to work on your leg action, as it does not compromise the head-neck-back relationship, it is the best practice for learning to breathe without shortening the neck.

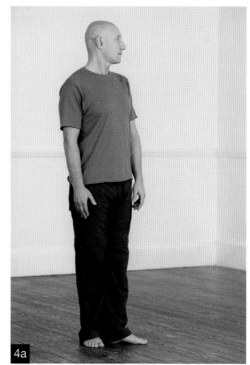
4a

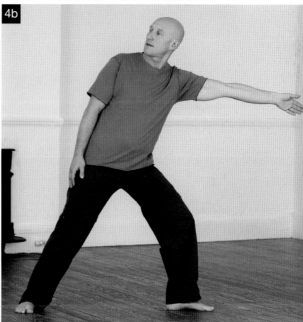
4b

- Start as in the previous practice. With your left arm leading, step forward, lower yourself into the water and drift off looking back and up (5a).
- Extend the left arm, angling it downward. Both ears should be submerged, your chin should be just breaking the surface and both eyes should be out of the water (5b).
- Alternately release the legs backward and press them forward, directing them upwards without breaking the surface.
- Continue for as long as is comfortable before repeating on the other side.

Remember *Allow the weight of the head to be supported by the water. The lead arm is connected with the primary control, which acts as a stable platform from which to balance. Keep the back arm soft and loose, creating space to breathe.*

Avoid *Do not arch the back, lift the shoulders, widen the legs, raise the lead arm or lift the head.*

6: Rotate to breathe

Stand upright in the pool, looking ahead, with the arms poised to begin the stroke. Open out the arms as you launch yourself on to your side and into the breathing position. This practice allows you to practise the transition of the head from facing forward to turning to the side, without the added complication of having to put the face in and out of the water.

It is an ideal way of learning to coordinate arm action, body rotation and head movement, so that you arrive at the breathing point in a

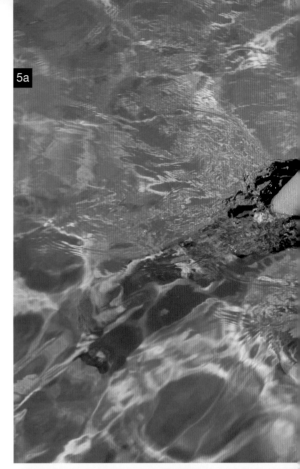

5a

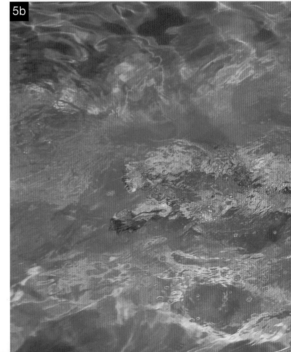

5b

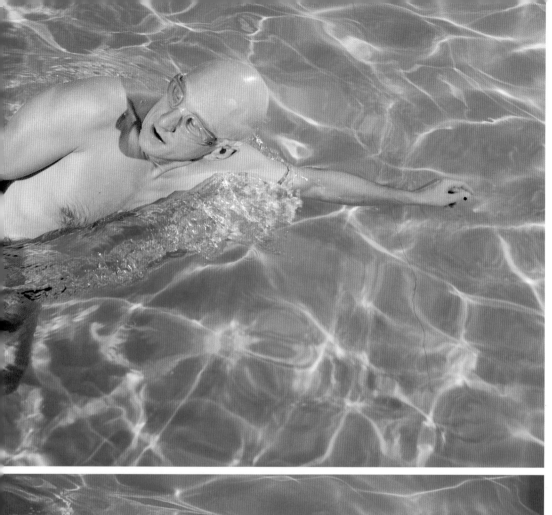

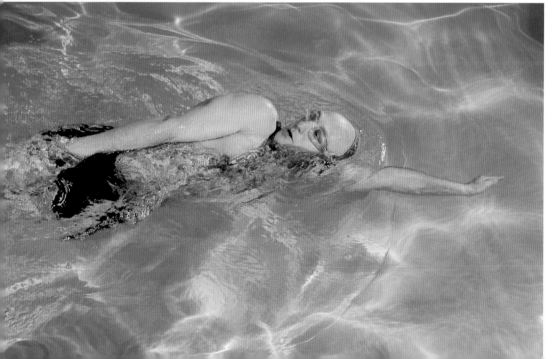

organized fashion. Dynamically rolling from an upright stance to lying on your side emphasizes the sensation of leading with the head, and feels like you are performing a diving header, in soccer terms.

- Begin in the opening stance and then take a small step with the right foot; both feet face forward.
- Extend the right arm and bring the left arm up and over into the salute position. Keep your weight evenly spread and your eyes looking ahead (6a).
- Without dropping your gaze, move up into the anchor phase, bringing your weight forward and the back foot up on tiptoe (6b).
- Exhale as you extend the left arm forward and allow the right arm to move towards the right hip, while the head and body dynamically rotate forward so that you are lying on your left side with your face out of the water (6c).
- Inhale gently and maintain this position for around ten seconds by working the legs (6d). Repeat the whole sequence four times before transferring to the other side.

Remember *Lead with the head and leave the neck free in the transitions. Concentrate on relaxed, gentle breathing through the mouth.*
Avoid *Do not pull the head back as you roll forward. Do not let the arm drift over the midline, or hunch the back shoulder.*

7. Rolling out to breathe
You have done this practice with a dry face: now you are now ready to progress to the

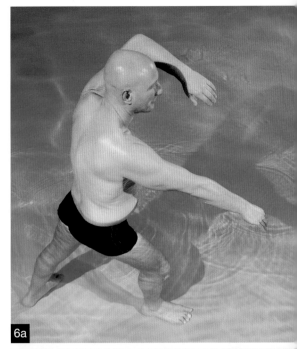
6a

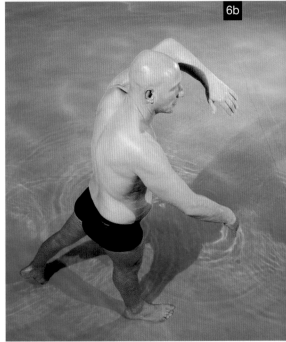
6b

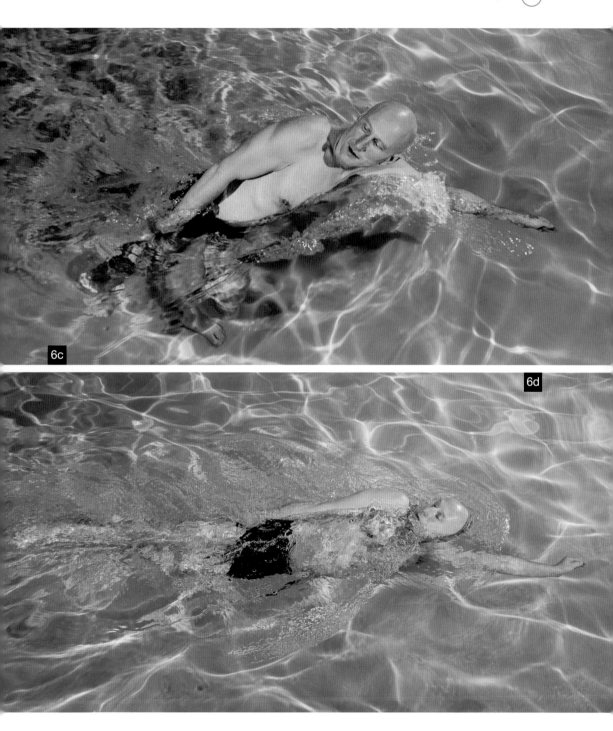

6c

6d

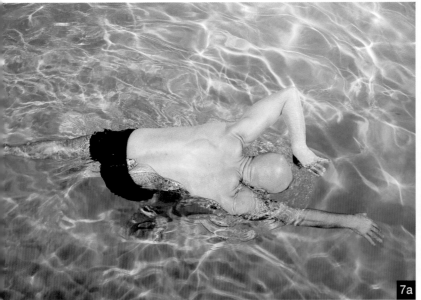
7a

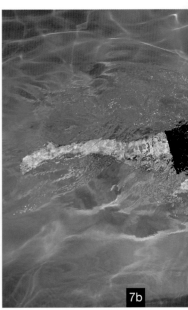
7b

transition between water and air. To prevent water getting up your nose, make sure you exhale in the transition between water and air.

- Drift off in the start position, with the right arm extended. Exhale gently, and maintain this position by using the leg action for a few seconds (7a).
- Flex the right wrist and elbow into the hook phase and direct them forward breathing out gently into the water (7b).
- Spiral and extend the left arm forward and down as the right arm holds the water, and the right hip and shoulder turn.
- Coordinate the head with the spiralling left arm so that it turns out of the water, ending up with the mouth and nose clear (7c).
- Breathe in gently through the mouth; use the legs to sustain a comfortable body position

on the side. Regain the feet and repeat on the other side.

Remember *Breathe out continuously in the transition between water and air. Direct the lead arm forward and down to give uplift.*
Avoid *Do not lift the head to breathe, turn the head after the back arm has completed the stroke, or inhale through the nose instead of the mouth.*

8. Two strokes – roll out

By integrating the turn made to breathe with a couple of full strokes, you get a clearer idea of the way your new breathing pattern fits into the stroke. Maintaining the breathing position at the end of the cycle will help you to inhale in a more relaxed manner and avoid the common tendency to snatch the breath.

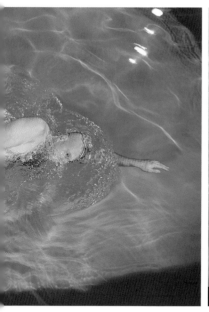

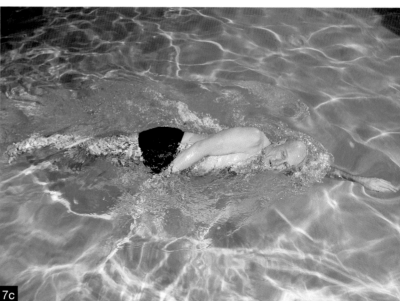

7c

- Leading with the right arm, swim two complete arm cycles with the face submerged. Look slightly ahead and start to exhale gently.
- At the start of the third cycle, roll outward by gently turning the head to the right, so the eyes, nose and mouth are clear of the water but the ears remain submerged.
- Allow the air to enter gently through the mouth; maintain this position by kicking on your side for six beats.
- Tuck up and regain your feet. After two complete stroke cycles, perform the sequence leading with the left arm.

Remember Maintain the same rhythm on breathing and non-breathing strokes. Focus on directing the lead arm forward rather than on the pulling arm.

Avoid Do not actively take a breath, inhale through the nose, or lift the head to inhale.

9. Returning the face
By working on the transition from the in-breath to the out-breath in isolation, you can learn to prevent the common mistake of dropping the lead arm before the head and recovering arm have entered the water. By maintaining the length of the lead arm, not only will you feel more control coming into the water, but you will also be able to achieve effective purchase.

- Drift off on your side, with the right arm leading and head turned left with the face out of the water. Maintain this position for six leg beats (9a).
- Gently raise the left arm and turn the neck to bring the face into the water as you rotate

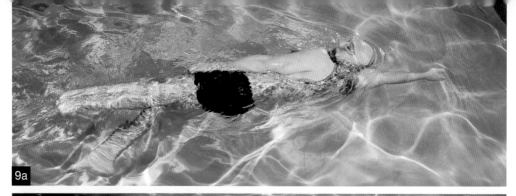

9a

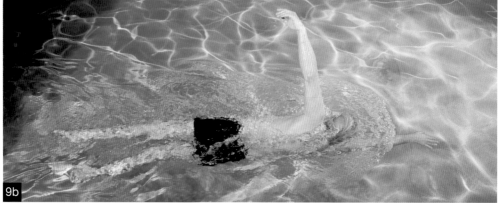

9b

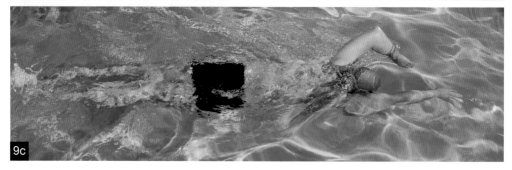

9c

the right arm (palm down) without dropping or shortening it (9b).

- Roll inwards until the hips and shoulders are almost parallel and the body is flat (9c).
- Maintain this central position for six beats before regaining your feet.
- Repeat the sequence on the other side.

Remember *The recovering arm should flow lightly through the air into the water.*

Avoid *Do not bear down heavily with the recovering arm, or drop the lead arm as the recovering arm is raised.*

10. Full-stroke bilateral breathing

Swim a continuous, steady front crawl, breathing every third or fifth stroke.

- Swing the recovering left arm; bend the right arm to hook and direct the recovering left arm forward and vice versa.
- During strokes where the face is submerged, breathe out gently when the arm holds the water, and a little more actively in the recovering phase.
- It's not necessary to rotate the body any further on the stroke that takes the face out of the water, than on strokes where the face remains submerged.

Remember *Keep a steady, even rhythm to the movement of the arms and legs. Hold the water with one arm and glide over it with the other, always lengthening and widening the back.*
Avoid *Do not hurry the pace of the arms in order to breathe. Do not gasp and lift the head to breathe, or drop the lead arm after inhaling as you roll back.*

One complete stroke

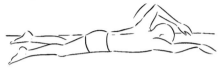

1. Centre the body with the eyes looking down, lead arm extended with the palm down and second arm in salute.

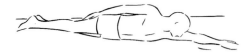

2. Flex the wrist of the lead arm and direct the elbow forward to anchor the water.

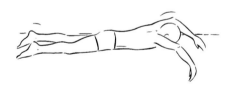

3. Direct the saluting arm forward to the handshake as the body dynamically rotates onto the side.

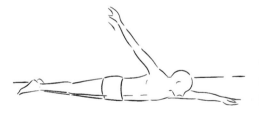

4. Direct the new lead arm forward as the recovering arm lengthens through the air, thumb leading, body centered.

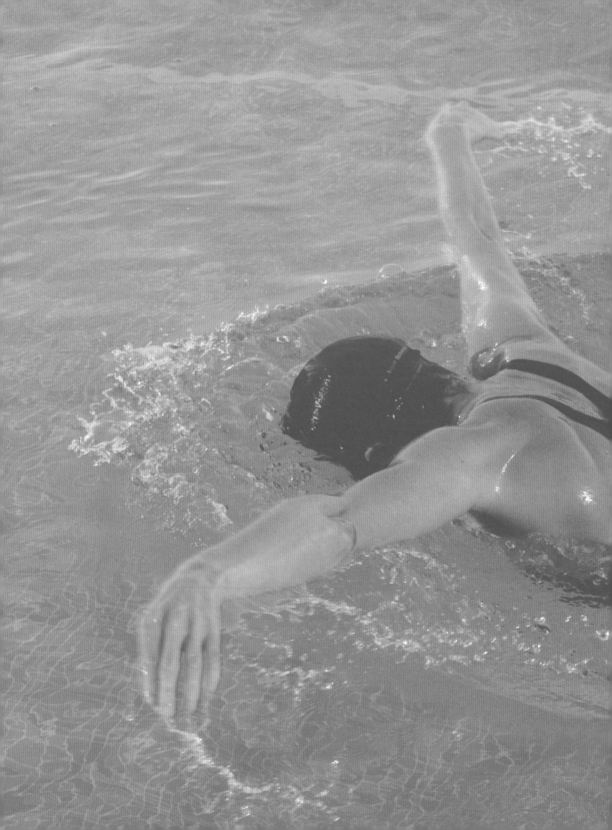

6

A SHAW WAY
TO FLY...

'Butterfly, it's brilliant! The natural undulating rhythm of butterfly allows one's whole being to flow in exhilarating harmony with the water.'

Vikki Harmer, registered Shaw Method teacher

Breaststroke to butterfly

Butterfly, the newest of the four traditional swimming styles, evolved from breaststroke. It was developed in the 1930s by US swimming coaches who were keen to make breaststroke faster. They found it frustrating that even though breaststroke generated a great deal of propulsive force, much of this was wasted during the underwater recovery phases. They made two major modifications: recovering the arms by moving them over the top, and experimenting with a dolphin-like leg action. This new version of the stroke was swum alongside classical breaststroke until the 1950s, when butterfly was finally designated a distinct stroke. Since then, butterfly has gone from strength to strength and is now the second quickest stroke.

Four-wheeled fly

In many ways, butterfly is the supreme stroke: a four-wheel drive stroke with equal propulsion coming from the upper and lower body, and where swimmer and water merge. Seen as the preserve of the strongest and fittest, swimming continuous butterfly seems completely out of reach to most people. Even amongst the most advanced fitness swimmers it is rare for anyone to be able to swim more than 200 metres (650ft) without feeling exhausted.

In this section you will discover that the butterfly is not necessarily more challenging than other strokes. As always in the Shaw Method, the key is to work intelligently with the water. Butterfly is an ideal opportunity to put your new relationship with the water to the test.

Without releasing tension and working with buoyancy you will struggle to progress.

The following lessons take you through a series of practices covering the core elements of the butterfly undulation, arm and leg actions, and integration of the breath. As in all strokes, only attempt the full stroke when you have consolidated the preliminary practices.

Shaw Method key features

Orientation Unlike conventional butterfly, where a powerful, dolphin-like leg kick is key to undulation, the head is key in the Shaw Method. The crown leads the body forward and down, with the eyes leading the body forward and up.

Arm action The arm recovery is low and wide, and connected to the movement of the hips and back. The slower, lighter arm recovery leading into a glide makes for a significantly more sustainable stroke. Beneath the surface, the focus is on holding the water to press the torso forward rather than pulling it back.

Leg action The two-beat, dolphin-like leg action is gentle and flowing, with the emphasis on pressing the legs down and allowing them to float up. This lighter action is less tiring and makes it easier to recover the arms.

Rhythm The hallmark of the Shaw Method butterfly is its steady, even rhythm and a strong sense of gliding through the water with the emphasis on allowing the water to lift the body.

Benefits

The continuous, wave-like action in butterfly is both energizing and calming. It mobilizes the spine, benefiting those with a stiff or tense back. People suffering from sciatica and other lower back conditions have experienced relief from learning the Shaw way to do butterfly. This benefit is in part the result of the strengthening effect that the undulating action has on the abdominals. The stroke helps to tone the arms and legs, and the wide overarm recovery broadens the back.

Risks and common mistakes

Alignment

1. Many people struggle to recover their arms, which often leads them to apply more effort, compounding the problem. The solution is to engage the hips and lower back; when the arms move backwards the hips sway forward and vice versa.

2. Many find it difficult to release the hips, making the arm and leg actions more difficult.

3. If you lift the head too high to breathe, it will cause the hips to sink too low. Keeping the head out of the water for too long impedes arm recovery, straining the neck and upper back.

Timing

1. Many have difficulty with coordination, attempting to push their hips and arms forward simultaneously.

2. If you breathe on every stroke it requires more effort and can lead to hyperventilation. Breathing on every second stroke is more efficient, providing more time to breathe out.

3. Many struggle to achieve the recommended cycle of two leg beats. In Shaw butterfly, we focus on the first leg beat and, by gliding at the end of the recovery, allow the second to occur naturally as a consequence of the undulation of the torso.

Propulsion

1. Many people overestimate the amount of effort required. Kicking too hard is not only tiring, but interrupts the flowing action of the arms. With the dolphin-like leg action it is important to press the legs down and allow them to float back up.

2. Another common stroke fault is to pull the arms straight back, rather than holding the water to propel the body forward. A higher, elbow-hooking action under the water improves purchase.

3. Many experience a build-up of tension in the arms and shoulders as a result of applying undue effort under the water. This can be addressed by releasing the arms as they approach the hips.

LESSON 1: UNDULATION

The overall impression of someone swimming the butterfly with style is a continuous, wave-like motion of the whole body. The movement of the arms and legs fades into the background as one witnesses this graceful action. In most swimming manuals, undulation is seen as a consequence of the dolphin-like leg action and the recovery of the arms. In the Shaw Method, the undulation is at the heart of the stroke, with the movement of the trunk making a significant contribution to overall propulsion, providing the foundation for both the arm and leg actions.

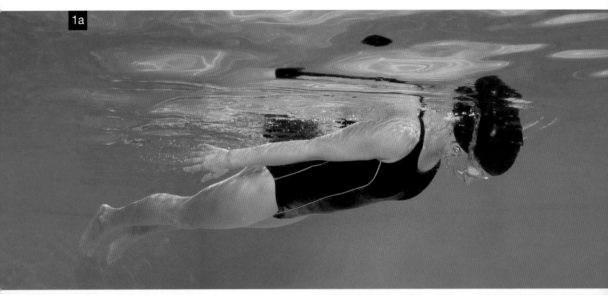

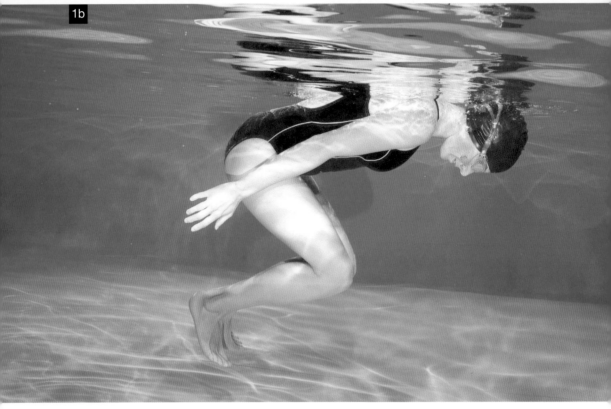

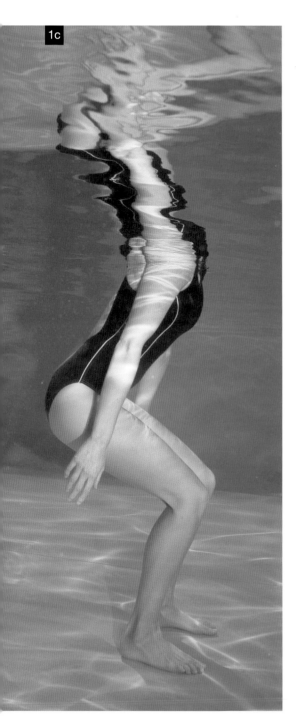

1c

Dolphin action

The legs remain together throughout and the movement flows through the hips, resembling a dolphin swimming along. Gliding with the knees released, a Shaw Method butterfly swimmer presses down with the upper body as the hips rise, then presses down with the legs, causing the upper body to be pushed to the surface.

This first lesson takes you though a series of practices in order to develop an effective dolphin action and master the art of undulation. A significant proportion of the overall propulsion is generated by the combined actions of the legs and the torso. It is important to be patient, as the wave-like motion is probably unlike anything you have done before. It may take a while before you can perform it with ease.

1. Body balance

The gliding phase of this practice develops your ability to balance without the support of the arms. This is an important skill in butterfly, the only stroke where both arms are simultaneously brought behind the body. Learning to regain the feet without the assistance of the arms develops your control of the core muscles, which is crucial to undulation.

- Inhale gently and step forward, arms by the sides. Bow forwards and start to exhale gently into the water.
- Without actively pushing, drift off into a glide with the eyes looking down and a sense of the crown leading the movement (1a).
- Maintain this stable position, without moving the limbs or trunk, for the count of four. Then

press the head down (1b) and tuck up to regain the feet without using the arms (1c).

● Repeat the above sequence leading off with the other leg.

Remember *Keep the neck free, and the shoulders and arms relaxed throughout.*
Avoid *Do not actively push off from the floor or pull the head back to regain the feet.*

2. Upright wave

This practice familiarizes you with moving the torso as one unit. It can been performed either floating upright in deep water or standing. The movement is assisted by the uplift of the water and the resistance offers useful feedback.

● Either take up the opening stance or tread water (see glossary).

● With palms facing to rear, tilt the upper body forward from the hips (2a), bend the knees slightly and if standing keep the heels in contact with the floor.

● The hips move forward and the upper back sways backwards as the arms gently sweep behind the body. If standing, move up on to tiptoes with eyes at eye level (2b).

● Repeat a number of times until the movement of arms and back feel integrated.

Remember *Move the body as one complete unit. Release the hips and relax the shoulders.*
Avoid *Do not arch the back or pull vigorously with the arms.*

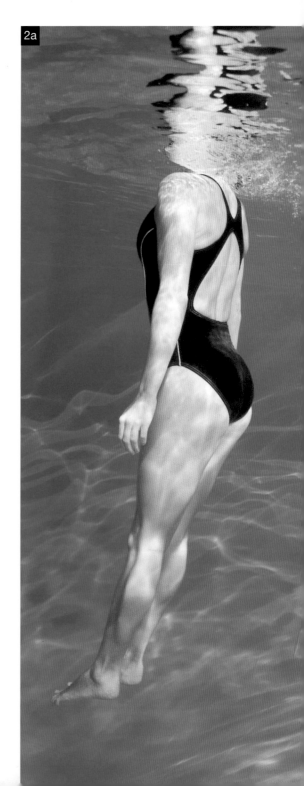
2a

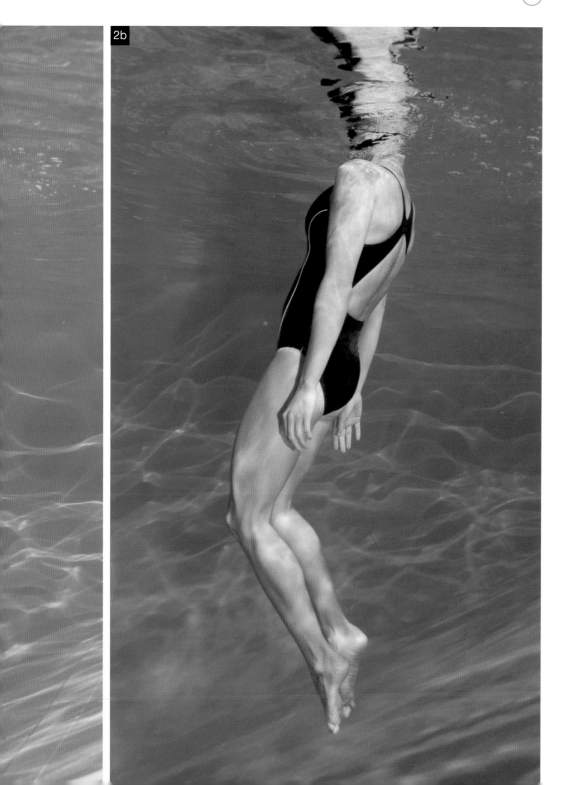

3. Wave – arms extended

This movement corresponds to the start of every stroke in butterfly. In this practice it is important to resist the temptation to pull the body down with the arms.

- Step forward. As the arms extend, bow the head and drift into a glide, eyes front, breathing out gently (3a).
- With your arms extended, press the chest down to allow the hips to rise, the crown of the head leading the body forward and slightly down. Ankles and knees loose (3b).
- Allow the legs to press down and the body to float up as you look ahead again. Look down to glide forward for a few seconds (3c) before regaining your feet.
- Move from a single wave into a series of waves. If you have difficulty doing more than one, press the chest forward as the body rises.

Remember *Move the body as a whole. The downward movement is active and the upward passive. Direct the undulating movement with your fingertips.*

Avoid *Do not stiffen the hips, over-bend the knees and lift the feet clear out of the water, pull the head back or hold your breath.*

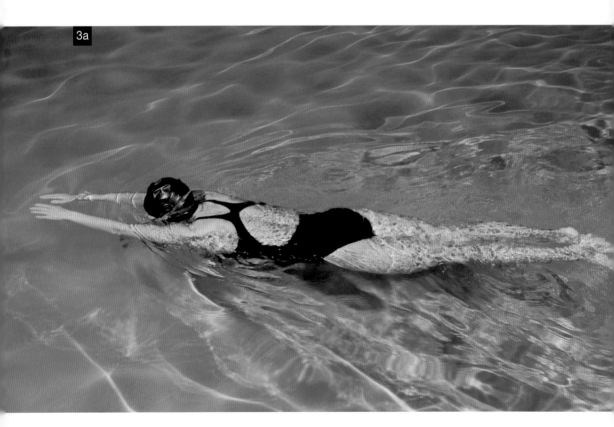

3a

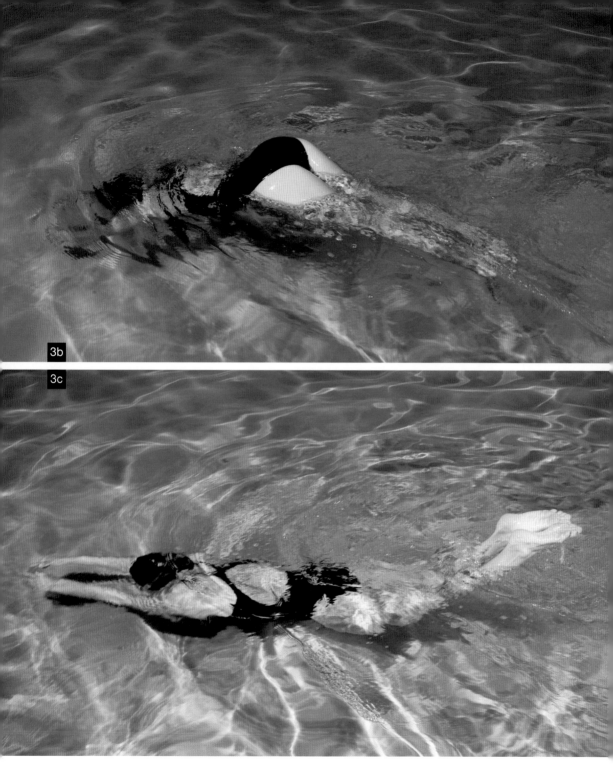

3b

3c

4. Wave – arms trailing

Both this and the previous practice give you the sensation of working the torso as one unit. Some find this practice easier; others find it harder. It is easier to be aware of the nodding action of the head in the undulation without the arms.

- Inhale gently, step forward with arms by the sides. Bow forwards, eyes looking ahead, and start to exhale gently (4a).
- Collapse the chest and actively press down, releasing the lower back so that the hips are driven upward as the legs extend (4b).

- Allow the upthrust of the water to lift the upper body as the knees bend and the hips move forward and down (4c). Regain your feet. Now attempt to link a series of undulations together.

Remember *Keep hands loose by your sides. Allow legs to lengthen and float up with the rest of the body. Enjoy the ebb and flow of this movement.*

Avoid *Do not arch the back unduly, poke the chin forward, over-bend the knees, lift the feet out of the water, or dive too deep.*

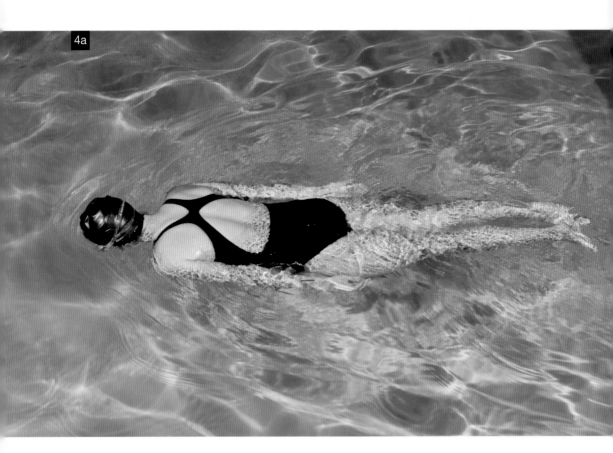
4a

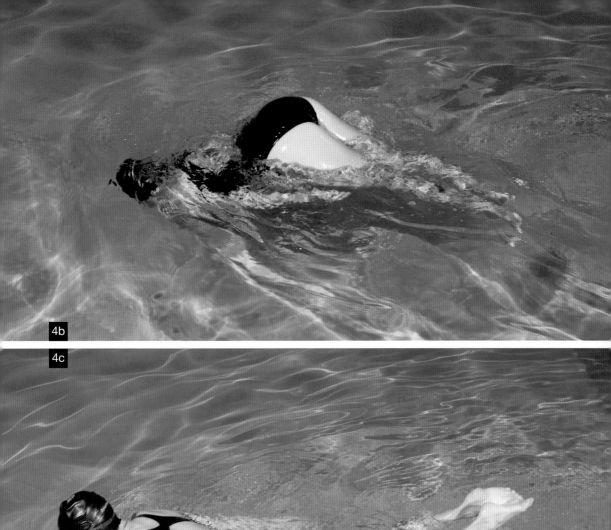

4b

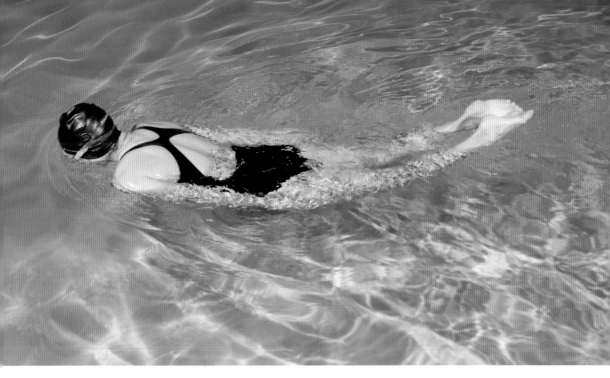

4c

LESSON 2: ARM ACTION

As discussed earlier, the arm action in butterfly is a consequence of the undulating movement of the torso. When the hips move forward and down, the arms sweep backwards (in the direction of the hips) and when the hips and back move backwards, the arms recover over the surface of the water. The symmetrical double arm action in butterfly can be broken down into four phases:

Extension The arms are directed forward and angled slightly down just within the width of the shoulders.

Lever The wrists are flexed and elbows bent.

Propulsive The holding phase, where the forearms actively pull the torso forward.

Recovery Both arms coast widely over the surface and lengthen into the extension phase.

The release into the recovery phase starts when both arms are still in the water; it is important not to pull too far backwards as this will tend to lock the arms. The recovery phase is often perceived as the most challenging, and many people waste unnecessary mental and physical effort trying to lift their arms over the water. This lesson teaches that when the other phases are working correctly, the recovery effectively happens by itself.

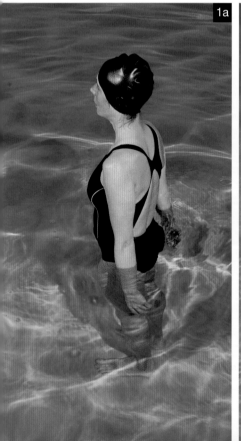

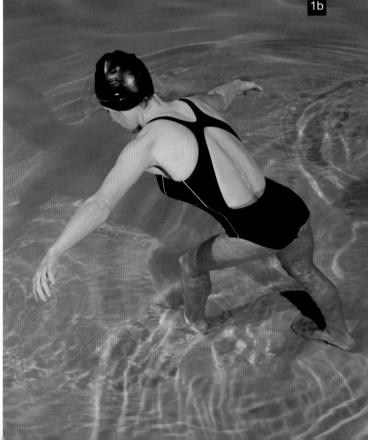

1. Spreading your wings

This action gives you a sense of how the movement of the back and pelvis promote an open and wide recovery action.

- Stand with your feet together, hips forward, knees slightly bent, and head gently tilted back so that the eyes look slightly up (1a).
- Open the shoulders and sweep the extended arms out to the side to just behind the hips, palms facing forward (1b). This promotes a sense of opening across the chest.
- Step forward with the left foot and start to exhale as you simultaneously sweep your arms over the surface of the water (1b).

Lengthen the back of the neck so the eyes are looking straight down. Whether or not your face ends up submerged depends on the depth of the pool (1c).

Remember *Keep most of your weight on the back foot as you step forward. Broaden the back across the shoulders as the arms sweep over the surface.*

Avoid *Do not narrow the back when the arms are in their initial position behind the hips. Do not allow the arms to become out of sync. Stifle the tendency to lead with the dominant arm.*

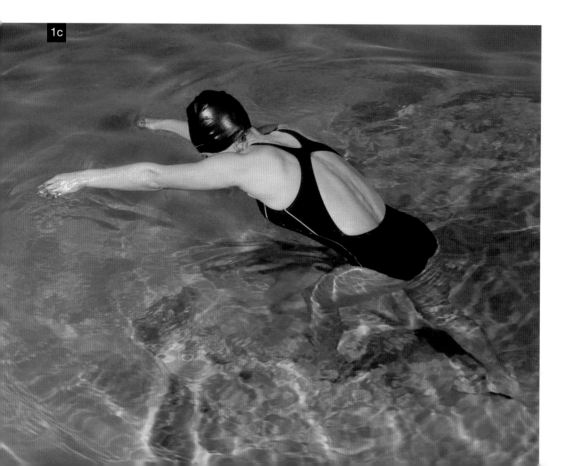

1c

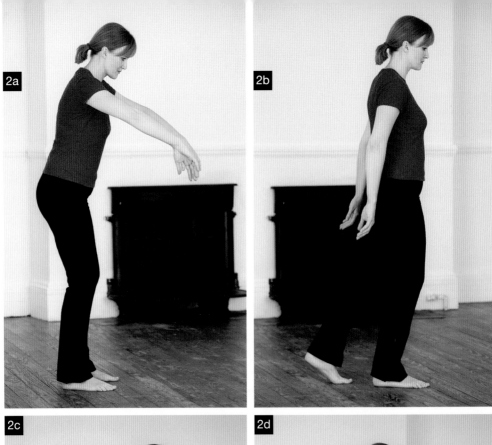

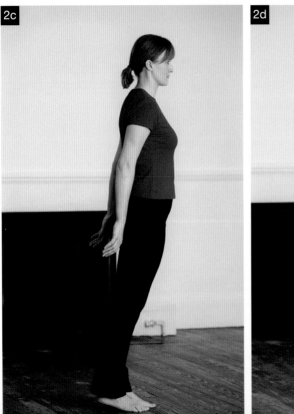

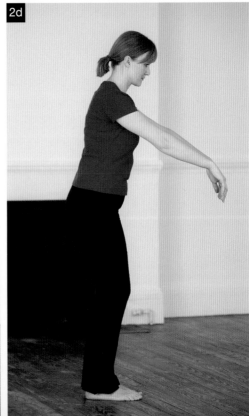

2. Stepping and sliding the arms

This practice can be performed in the water or on dry land, and helps you appreciate how the arms and hips combine to produce forward momentum. On dry land, the arm recovery is very straightforward. With the resistance of water, it is more of a challenge, which further highlights the importance of a gentle recovery.

- Bend the knees and allow your torso to incline forward as you lengthen along the spine (2a). Leading with the wrists, slide the arms forward until they are fully extended and direct your gaze towards the floor.
- Flex the hands and release the elbows as you prepare the forearms as if to take hold of the water, with weight evenly distributed on both feet.
- Push the hips forward and gently bend the back (2b) as you take two small steps forward (2c).
- In one continuous action, incline the torso and extend the arms forward (2d). Repeat the whole sequence five or six times.

Remember *The arms act as levers to draw the torso forward, actively pressing the air out as the torso inclines forward. Inhale as the hips thrust forward and arms move back.*
Avoid *Do not move the arms without changing the position of the hips. Do not over-arch, or hyper-extend the spine.*

3. Soaring

This practice involves pressing the body down and pulling it back up with the arms. This is one of the most important of the butterfly practices, as it establishes the overall rhythm of the stroke and highlights the relationship between the dolphin-like leg action and the underwater phase of the arms.

- Launch off into a glide with your arms extended, knees slightly bent and eyes looking in the direction of travel; breathe out gently into the water.
- Nod your head as you actively straighten the legs and press the body downward whilst maintaining the length and direction of both arms (3a).
- Look ahead, gently tilting the head backwards, and as the body starts to float

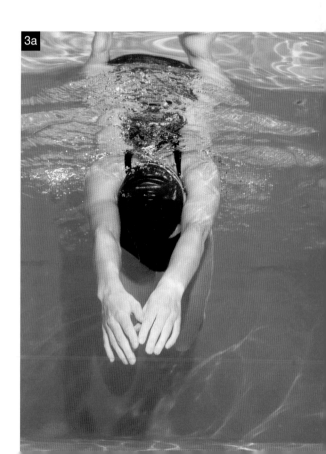
3a

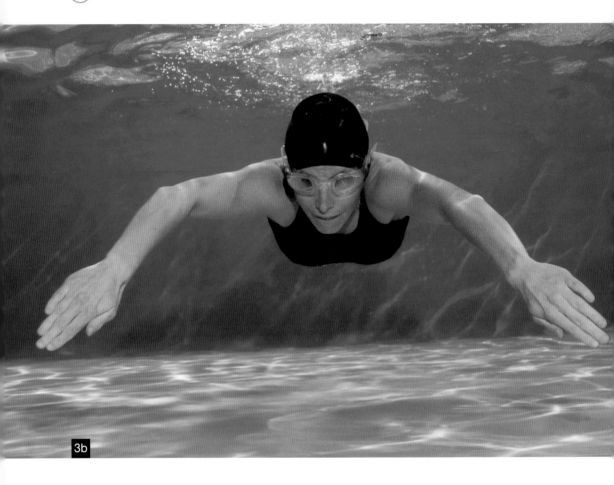

3b

up, open the arms, flex the hands and bend the elbows (3b).

- Hold on to the water and allow the head to lead the body forward and up to the surface (3c). Do not be concerned if this brings your face out of the water.
- Remain with your arms by your side, eyes looking ahead and knees bent, until you stop moving forward, at which point tuck to regain the feet with your arms by your sides.

Remember *Flex the hands and bend the elbows. Release the arms towards the waist as you press the hips toward the floor.*
Avoid *Do not go too deep by using the arms to pull you down rather than to assist elevation.*

4. Wave revisited

This revision practice reconnects you to the undulation which is at the heart of the stroke. This combination of the extended and trailing arm undulations serves as a timely reminder not to overwork the arms. It also gives an

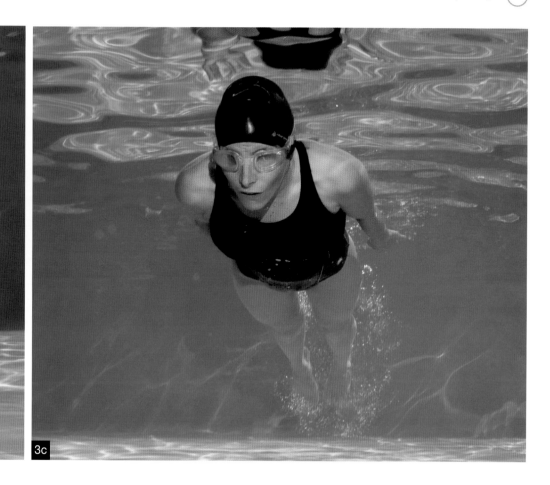

3c

opportunity to experiment with applying a major and minor dolphin action.

- Exhaling gently, glide with the arms extended, knees bent and eyes looking slightly ahead. Actively press down with the head to hollow the chest and release the lower back so that the hips are driven upward. Thrust with the legs as they extend allowing the head and fingertips to lead your upper body down.
- Look up and direct the chest and arms forward as the upper body travels towards the surface.
- As the body starts to float up open the arms, flex the hands and bend the elbows. Gently tilt the head backwards. Hold onto the water and move forward with the chest as you press the body up towards the surface.
- Instead of pausing as in the previous practice, undulate again but with the arms trailing by the sides. As with the arms extended, perform a second lighter and smaller undulation before regaining the feet.

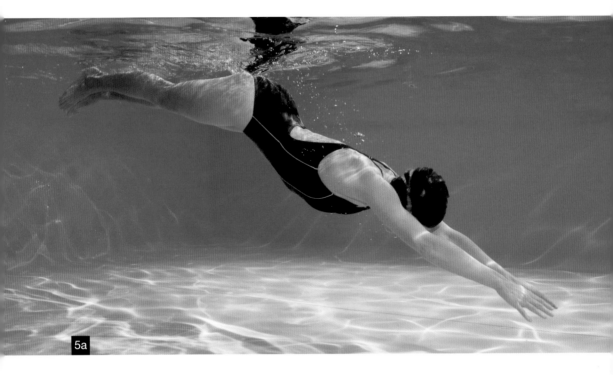

5a

5. Breastafly

This practice helps counter the common mistake of overemphasizing the action of lifting the arms clear of the water while not paying attention to what happens below. Because this form of recovery creates resistance, it encourages the pattern of making a soft recovery, which is important in the full stroke – a positive side effect of the practice.

- Inhale gently and launch smoothly into a glide, with both arms extended, the head slightly tilted back, eyes looking ahead.
- With the arms still extended, bow the head to push the upper body down towards the floor (5a).
- Flex the wrists and bend the elbows to take hold of the water (5b), and thrust the hips and chest forward as you propel yourself towards the surface.
- Draw the hands together in front of chest with the eyes looking down (5c).
- Slide the arms forward as if you were performing a breaststroke arm recovery.
- Repeat the whole sequence a second time and regain the feet.

Remember *Accelerate forward and down with the lower body and then forward and up with the upper body, using the recovery to balance.* **Avoid** *Do not lift the arms out of the water. Do not exhale forcefully as this will make you sink.*

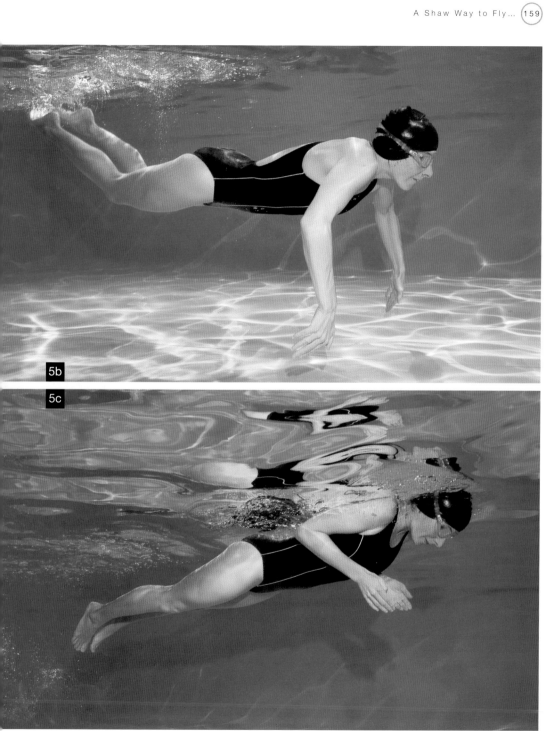

5b

5c

6. Arm action with feet on the ground

Standing stationary, follow the same sequence of arm and body movements as in the second practice, but instead of performing an underarm recovery, bring the arms over the top as the hips sway back. Being upright, with the face permanently clear of the water, it is easier to learn the rhythm of the stroke as you can continue the movement many times without needing to stop for a breath.

- Extend the arms forward, leading with the wrists, and allow the hips to release back as the upper body sways forward. Keep the legs bent with the heels on the floor (6a).
- Draw the arms back as the hips incline forward and the weight shifts on to the balls of the feet, knees slightly bent (6b).
- In one continuous movement, leading with the tips of the little fingers, start to swing the arms (6c) up and over the top (6d).

Remember *The overarm recovery is a consequence of the movement of the hips and arms beneath the surface.*
Avoid *Do not push at any point during the cycle, particularly when the arms are behind you, as it makes the arms feel heavier in the recovery.*

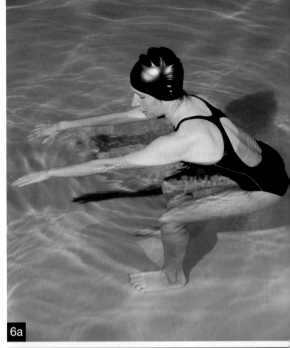
6a

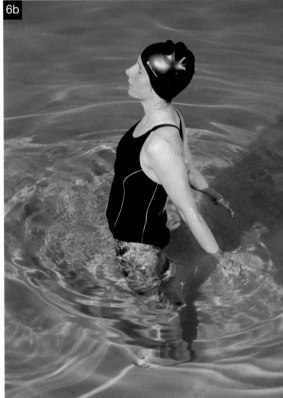
6b

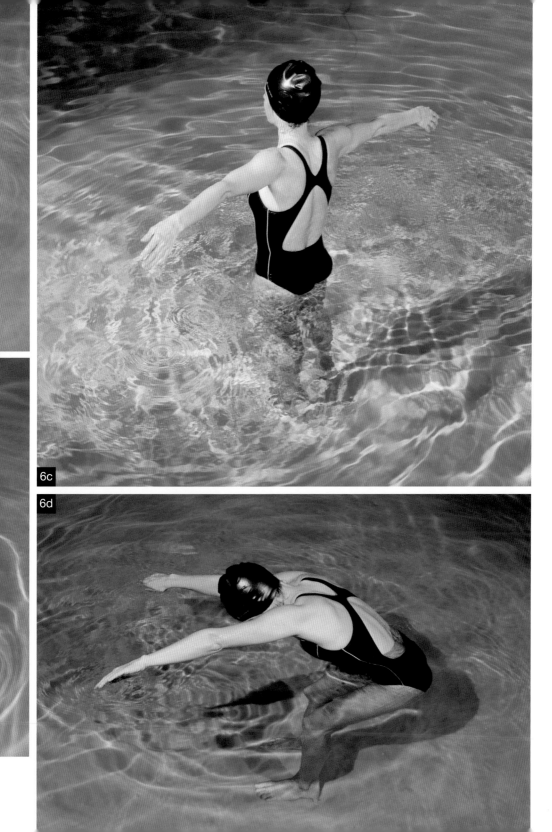

6c

6d

7. Complete arm action

After practising all the individual elements of the stroke, you are now ready to put it all together. A pause at the end of the cycle gives you the opportunity to discover the second dolphin beat, which often gets left out in continuous butterfly swimming.

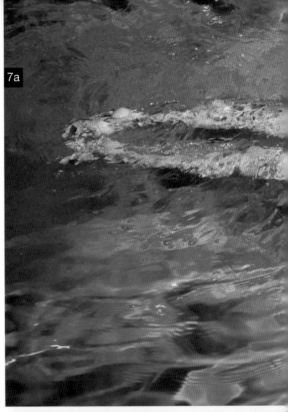

7a

- From a glide, perform one full stroke with the face in the water and an overarm recovery (7a–d).
- At the end of the cycle, maintain the length of the arms and relax. You will notice a second small wave through the body. This second wave is a consequence of the arm recovery and should be allowed to happen by itself rather than actively creating it.
- Glide for three or four seconds, then undulate without shortening the arms and regain the feet.

Remember *Release the pressure in the arms when they pass the thigh.*
Avoid *Do not pull the arms beyond the hips or rush the arms forward in the recovery.*

8. Two complete strokes

Now you have integrated the torso, arms and legs with face submerged for one stroke, you can progress to performing this action a couple of times. Swimming with the face in the water helps establish flow and rhythm without the pressure of having to breathe.

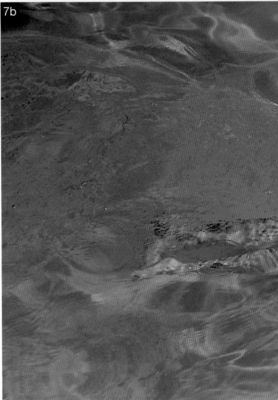

7b

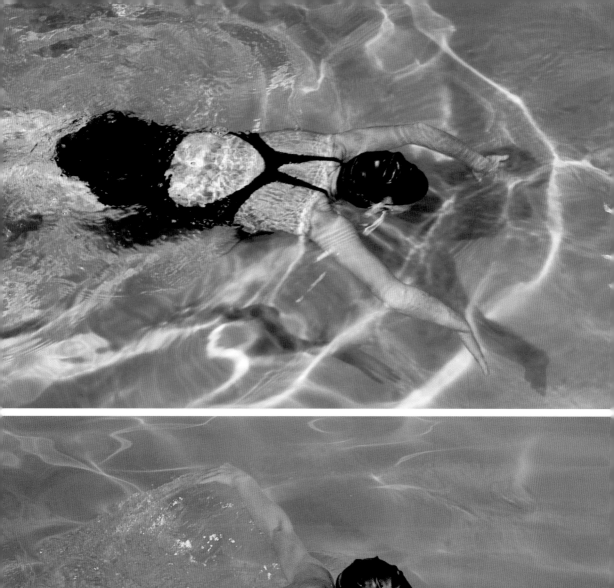

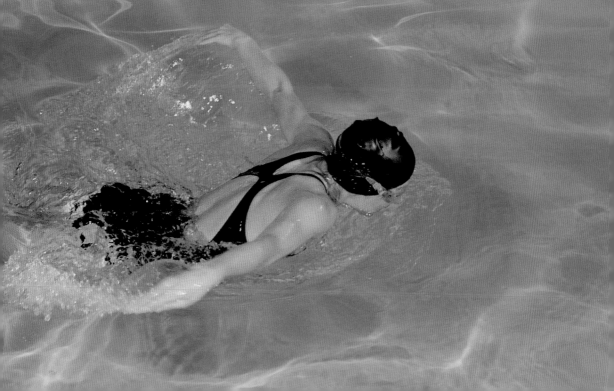

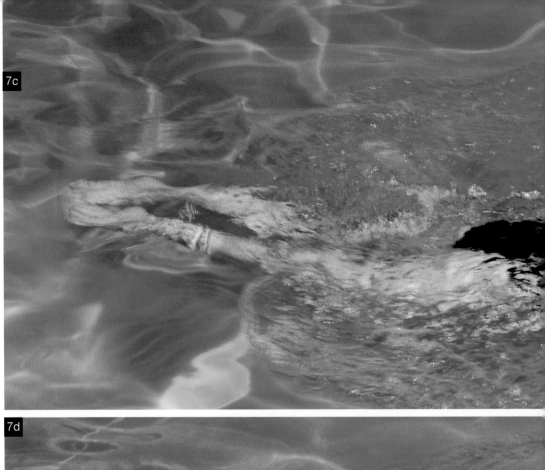

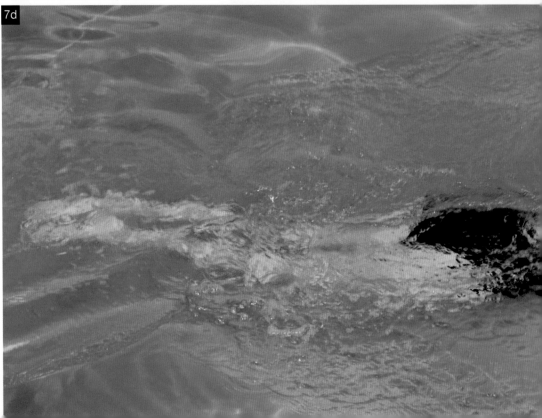

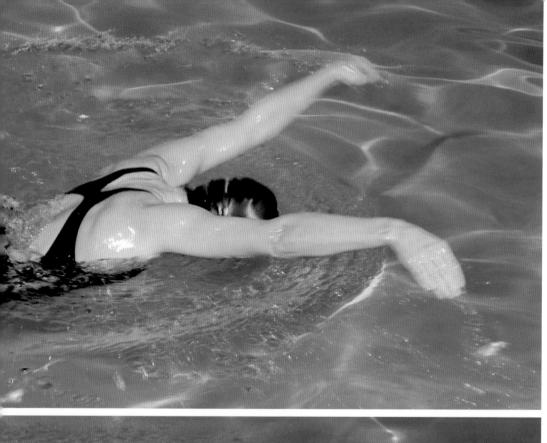
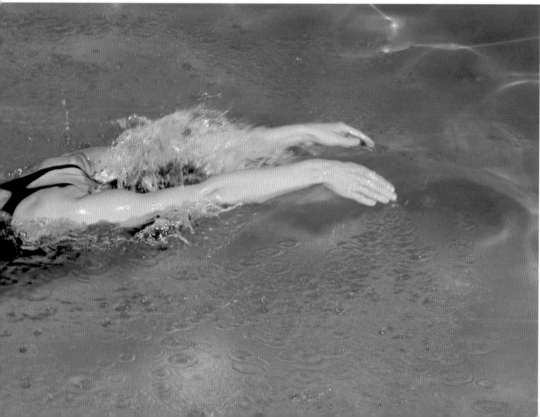

LESSON 3: INTEGRATING THE BREATH

Issues concerning breathing are a major cause of anxiety for those wishing to master butterfly, and three of the most serious stroke faults are rooted in a lack of confidence.

Struggling to get the face out of the water to breathe leads many people to lift their heads too high, which not only wastes energy but also creates excessive drag as the lower body is forced down. This also leads to the tendency, discussed in the other strokes, to actively inhale, which can give rise to hyperventilation. Unease about breathing also causes swimmers to keep their faces out of the water for too long. Pulling the head back during the recovery of the arms makes this action more of an effort and strains the neck.

Breathing with ease

In butterfly, as with the other strokes, explosive breathing is detrimental. However, the intense and explosive way in which most people approach the stroke means that forceful exhalations are unavoidable.

This can be countered by slowing down and relaxing. You will feel less desperate to take a breath and consequently able to negotiate the transition between water and air more fluently. Efficient breathing entails allowing the head to lift gently rather than snatching it out of the water, which is a sure way to give yourself a whiplash injury! The head moves wiith each undulation, and all that is necessary for the face to break the surface is to continue this movement a little further.

Until recently, swimming coaches generally required swimmers to breathe every other stroke. It was believed that even a slight lift of the head reduced streamlining and speed, but then came Michael Phelps, butterfly world record holder and Olympic champion, who breathes on every stroke. Experiment with different breathing patterns and find out what works best for you. Whatever you choose, always exhale at the end of the recovery; to do it any earlier will put your head out of sync with the undulating action of the rest of the body.

In an attempt to reduce resistance, some butterfly swimmers have even started turning their head to the side to keep it as low as possible. I find this way of breathing problematic, as when my head turns I feel that the rest of my body wants to follow. But feel free to try it out for yourself: my reluctance may be the result of habitual patterns carried over from the front crawl.

1. Breathing – feet on the ground

Practise coordinating your breathing with the arm action in shallow water.

- Stand with your feet together, arms extended and eyes looking straight ahead.
- Exhale as you press the hips forward and draw the arms to your sides, allowing the knees to bend. Notice how, at the end of this pull phase, you spontaneously feel like inhaling (1a).
- Resume the exhalation as the arms swing over, leading with the little finger (1b).
- Continue the practice for six cycles; pause.

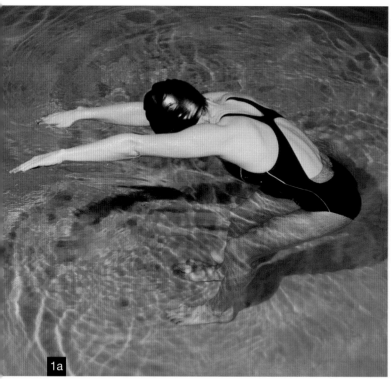

1a

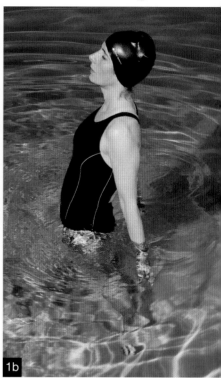

1b

Remember *Sway the hips and allow the exhalation to follow the recovery phase naturally.*
Avoid *Do not breathe in reverse, i.e. inhale on the recovery and exhale at the end of the pull phase.*

2. Breathing for butterfly on land

Now practise coordinating your breathing with the arm action on dry land.

Although you are standing, the fact that in this practice you move forward as the arms perform their propulsive phase gives you a good sense of the stroke's rhythm and further integrates the timing of breathing learned in the previous practice.

- Perform the same sequence of movements as in the previous practice, but instead of keeping the feet still, step forward in dynamic holding phase.
- As the arms recover over the surface, keep the feet still.

Remember *The torso is propelled forward and the arms flow lightly through the air.*
Avoid *Do not over-arch the back or keep it too straight. Do not tense the arms.*

3. Two complete strokes, breathing on the second one

Combine poise, power, ease and fluidity.

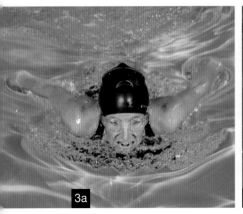

3a

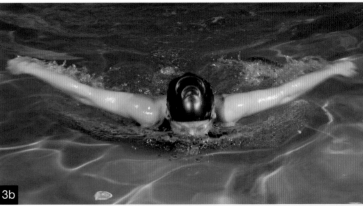

3b

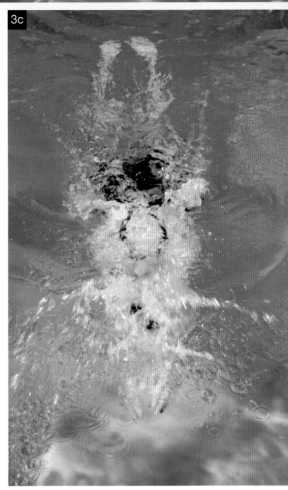

3c

- Glide with relaxed arms extended to a width that is a little narrower than shoulder width.
- Undulate forward and down, release the legs so that they are slightly bent and then actively press them down to start the elevation of the body towards the surface.
- Use the arms to pull the body towards the surface, allowing the eyes to look ahead but without bringing them out of the water.
- Release the arms as they pass your thighs; at this point begin to press the chest forward and release the hips so that the arms can flow through the air easily. The arms enter the water rotated slightly outwards.
- Glide until you feel a second smaller undulation pass through you.
- Repeat the same sequence as for the first movement, raising the eye level more during the arms' propulsive phase so that the mouth breaks the surface (3a) and you inhale gently.
- Bring the face swiftly back into the water and start to exhale (3b) as the arms recover over the surface (3c).

Remember *The first stronger leg beat occurs when the arms are extended, the second during the recovery.*

Avoid *Do not apply too much force with the legs, creating a big splash.*

One complete stroke

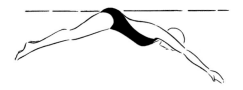

1. Start with arms forward, eyes looking slightly forward and knees released.

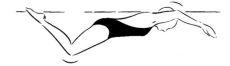

2. Press the head down. Hips move up as the legs extend, eyes down.

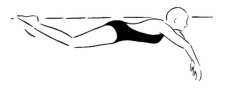

3. Raise the head, bring the eyes up, flex the wrist and bend the elbows as hips start to move forward.

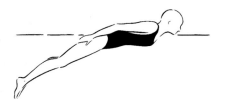

4. With eyes leading hold the water, press the chest and hips forward, hands relaxed.

FINAL WORD

I suggested earlier that fitness objectives need to be put to one side until you can move well in the water. The tendency to drift back to old habits is greatest when swimming the full stroke, so continue working with the Shaw Method practices. They will keep you mindful of the core features of each stroke and many of them, as well as promoting good form, can be incorporated into your exercise routine. For example, the front crawl practice where the body rotates and the arms perform an underwater recovery can be developed into a good cardiovascular workout by turning the head to breathe.

As each stroke has its own essential character and rhythm it is beneficial to swim a variety. However, avoid chopping and changing too often as it takes time settle into each stroke. I, personally, find it takes me at least ten minutes to get accustomed to a stroke's subtleties before I am ready to move on. One of the best ways to assimilate this work is to share your experience with others. For example, if you are struggling to co-ordinate the arms and legs in breaststroke, it is useful to offer to teach someone else an aspect of the stroke that you have already grasped. Apart from boosting morale this will deepen your own understanding.

Many are enticed by the prospect of swimming freely in a natural environment, for others this has long been an unattainable dream. Whatever your starting point, having invested time and effort mastering the art of swimming, the allure of open water is likely to be very strong. By all means pursue this ambition and enjoy the sense of freedom that it brings but get to know the new environment and take care. Simon Murie of SwimTrek, a channel swimmer and seasoned open water guide, never swims more than 100 meters out to sea unaccompanied. Others may be drawn to training for some form of competition such as master swimming or triathlon. This is a great way to reap the rewards of your mindful practice and meet other swimming enthusiasts. Remember to pay attention to good form and do not get too distracted by results.

Shaw Method essentials

Below is a useful summary of the principles underpinning the Shaw Method learning process.

● The maintenance of a balanced head-neck-back (HNB) relationship is key. Whatever is happening with the rest of your body is secondary. The HNB affects your swimming performance more than anything else, particularly when it comes to the transition between water and air.

- Remember that before every propulsive movement there is a vital non-propulsive action. Undue effort in the non-propulsive phase undermines the ability to achieve an effective purchase on the water.
- Give attention to directing yourself forward rather than pulling backwards. This can also be a metaphor for the rest of your life.
- Efficient swimming is more about learning to let go than it is about doing more. Be patient with yourself and remember that trying to get it right is often the biggest impediment to the learning process. Be gentle with yourself as changing your relationship with water can stir up powerful emotions.
- Always co-ordinate breathing with the stroke. Breath-holding is not recommended!
- Your swimming will develop better when backed up by work out of the water. Dry land practices are a remarkably effective way of establishing new patterns of movement.
- Think in terms of phases rather than positions. In order to learn the strokes it has been necessary to break the movements down into their essential parts. When swimming continuously, flow rhythmically from one phase to the next.
- Cultivate a mindful approach and learn to interact artistically with the water. Stop working against the water and start swimming with it.
- Don't judge your performance by others' standards. Remember swimming is an adventure into the unknown, not a struggle to get things right.
- Finally, remember to be creative, have fun and explore the water. Don't be dogmatic, there is more than one way to cross a river. My own swimming and the Method continue to evolve.

Equipment

Swimming is accessible to all and does not require much equipment. It is worth splashing out on a decent costume and a good pair of goggles. Avoid suits that trap air or water and for woman make sure there is ample space for the arms to move freely. From the wide range of swimming eyewear available I find Aqua Sphere offer great panoramic vision and are easy to adjust. In the early stages of learning the Shaw Method it is necessary to work at a measured pace which in cooler water can lead to physical and mental tension. Light non-buoyant thermal tops, available at dive shops, are great for maintaining a comfortable temperature.

Art of Swimming learning resources

The Art of Swimming: a new direction with the Alexander Technique
Steven Shaw and Armand D'Angour (1997, Ashgrove Press). This book provides a valuable introduction of how to apply Alexander Technique principles to swimming.
Art of Swimming DVD explores the benefits of swimming particularly as the ideal remedy for stress. Filmed in the Red Sea, this film is an inspirational adventure into the art of swimming.
Shaw Method Steps VHS This video, featuring individual and partner practices, shows a series of steps for breaststroke, front crawl and backstroke. It is ideal for both water confident swimmers and teachers wishing to view core Shaw Method practices.
Laminated pool cards with our unique series of progressive stroke-by-stroke practices.
There is also a range of stroke specific DVD's that combine footage of dry land practices with clear underwater and above water sequences. These include *Learn to Crawl Again*, *Time to Fly*, *Breaststroke with Ease* and *Better your Backstroke*.

Lessons in the Art of Swimming

Although this book and the various learning resources are very useful there is no substitute for the experience of learning with a registered Shaw Method teacher (RSMT). Art of Swimming offers a comprehensive package of learning opportunities. These include one to one lessons, weekly classes, day workshops, residential courses, corporate events and swimming holidays. Lessons take place in a variety of venues, which have been selected to provide a calm, focused learning environment. To find out more visit www.artofswimming.com, or call +44 (0) 20 8446 9442.

Learning the Alexander Technique

Shaw Method work is best combined with lessons in the Alexander Technique. The teacher will use explanation and a guiding touch to help you rediscover balance and ease within yourself. Through experience and observation, you learn to develop your body awareness, how you create tension and how to prevent or release it. Although your teacher is unlikely to be a specialist in working with people in the water, your new skill and understanding will positively impact on your approach to swimming. Visit www.stat.org.uk to find out more.

GLOSSARY

Bilateral breathing Breathing on both sides in front crawl as opposed to unilateral breathing, which is on just one side. In terms of good use, a bilateral pattern is clearly preferable as it promotes symmetry.

Breaststroker's knee Most knee injuries are related to the use of the whip kick. 'Breaststroker's knee' is the result of repetitive stress to the Medial Collateral Ligament.

Drag This impedes motion; the level of drag is determined by the degree of resistance created by an object's size, shape or orientation. This is one of the reasons why a bus moves more slowly than a sports car and why the rotated orientation in crawl is more streamlined than the flatter positioning of breaststroke.

Explosive breathing A common practice in competitive swimming where breath is held and then blown out forcefully just prior to inhalation.

Holding the water The idea of using the arms as levers to transport the torso forward rather than the common tendency of pulling back. Front arm crawl action is similar to pulling along a rope.

Hyperventilation Unusually deep or rapid breathing often caused by anxiety or habit, leading to a feeling of breathlessness and sometimes faintness.

Screw Kick An uneven breaststroke leg action in which one foot is turned in and the other turned out throwing one side of the pelvis forward with each kick; it strains the sacro-iliac joint and is potentially injurious.

Sculling A motion employing rotational hand movements often in a figure of eight, which can be performed on the back, front or vertically. It helps develops a 'feel for the water' important to all strokes.

Swimmer's shoulder (tendonitis) An injury that develops through misuse of the shoulder joint (rotator cuff) resulting in inflammation and pain. The body rotation and relaxed recovery employed in Shaw Method crawl reduce the incidence of this.

Treading water A skill requiring a combination of limb movements in order to remain upright in the water without submersing the face. There are various ways of treading water with good alignment which do not require much effort.

Trickle breathing Gradual exhalation with the face in the water.

Tumble turn A spin and underwater push off from the wall used in back and front crawl, incorporating a half forward somersault and twist. Tumble turns allow you to swim laps continuously without losing rhythm.

Undulation A wave-like action of the body employed in breaststroke and butterfly.

INDEX

Further Reading

Body Learning: An Introduction to the Alexander Technique Michael Gelb (Aurum Press, 1994)

Body Mind Mastery: Creating success in sport and life Dan Millman (New World Library, 1999)

Flow M Csikenthmihaly (Harper & Row, 1990)

Haunts of the Black Masseuse Charles Sprawson (Vintage, 1993)

Indirect Procedures: A musicians guide to the Alexander Technique Pedro de Alcantara (Clarendon, 1997)

In Praise of Slow Carl Honore (Orion, 2004)

Master the Art of Running Malcolm Balk & Andrew Shields (Collins & Brown, 2006)

Swimming for the Health of it E Maglischo & C Ferguson Brenan (Mayfield 1985)

The Owner's Guide to the Body Roger Golten (Thorsons, 1999)

The Alexander Technique – as I see it Patrick Macdonald (Rahula Books, 1989)

The Art of Swimming: A new direction using the Alexander Technique S Shaw & A D'Angour (Ashgrove, 1996)

The Use of the Self: F Mathias Alexander (Gollancz, 1935,1985)

Total Immersion Terry Laughlin & John Delves; (Simon & Schuster, 1996)

Waterlog: A Swimmers Journey Through Britain Roger Deakin (Vintage, 2000)